# JUMPSTART
# TO
# SKINNY

# JUMPSTART
# TO
# SKINNY

*The Simple 3-Week Plan for*

*Supercharged Weight Loss*

# BOB HARPER

*with Greg Critser*

BALLANTINE BOOKS

NEW YORK

This book proposes a program of diet and exercise recommendations for the reader to follow. However, you should consult a qualified medical professional (and, if you are pregnant, your ob/gyn) before starting this or any other fitness program. Please seek your doctor's advice before making any decisions that affect your health or extreme changes in your diet, particularly if you suffer from any medical condition or have any symptom that may require treatment. As with any diet or exercise program, if at any time you experience any discomfort, stop immediately and consult your physician.

Copyright © 2013 by Bob Harper Enterprises

Published in the United States by Ballantine Books, an imprint of The Random House Publishing Group, a division of Random House, Inc., New York.

BALLANTINE and colophon are registered trademarks of Random House, Inc.

Photographs by Adam Rindy

LIBRARY OF CONGRESS CATALOGING-IN-PUBLICATION DATA
Harper, Bob.
Jumpstart to skinny: the simple 3-week plan for supercharged
weight loss / Bob Harper; with Greg Critser.
pages   cm
Includes bibliographical references and index.
ISBN 978-0-345-54510-7
eBook ISBN 978-0-345-54511-4
1. Reducing exercises. 2. Weight loss. 3. Reducing diets—recipes.
I. Critser, Greg. II. Title.
RA781.6.H357 2013   613.2'5—dc23   2012051372

Printed in the United States of America on acid-free paper

www.ballantinebooks.com

2 4 6 8 9 7 5 3 1

First Edition

Book design by Caroline Cunningham

*For Karl*

# CONTENTS

PART II:

# THE JUMPSTART DAY-BY-DAY REGIMEN

PART III:

# THE JUMPSTART MOVES

PART IV:

# THE JUMPSTART RECIPES

# INTRODUCTION

Not long ago I got an urgent call from one of my celebrity clients.

"You've got to help me, Bob," she said. "I'm performing in three weeks and I want to go on stage without *hiding my body behind my guitar!*"

Like so many of us, she'd put off getting in shape and losing weight in the months leading up to her big show, and now she needed some fast-acting advice to get her on stage feeling confident, comfortable, and looking like the rock star she is.

If you've read my book *The Skinny Rules,* you know that she could have followed those nonnegotiable principles for getting to thin a long time ago and she wouldn't be in the fix she found herself in now. But it hadn't yet been published and she didn't have a lot of time anyway. She needed me to whip her into shape ASAP.

I get it: having a goal and a deadline is the motivation that many of us need to make a change, get off the couch, get our noses out of the fridge, and get ourselves back onto the path of a healthy (and slimming) life.

"I have good news," I replied. "You're now very motivated—you have a very specific goal and you're on a very tight, specific timetable. I can work with that. I have a plan that will put you on stage looking and feeling like a knockout. You have to follow this plan for the next three weeks. You have to follow it to the letter. You need to buckle down. And I promise that you'll love the way you look and feel for the big show. And I promise, too, that you'll want to keep it up afterwards, and for that you'll transition to *The Skinny Rules*. Are you in?"

Her response? "Hell yes!"

My rock star client's looming performance conjured the same anxiety many of us experience while preparing for, say, a wedding: Will my dress make me look fab, or fat? Will my tux look form-fitting, or chub-containing?

Or a reunion: Will all those classmates envy or pity me?

Or an upcoming beach vacation: Can I get away with a bikini or a Speedo (although I'm a board shorts kind of guy), or should I just stay in the hotel room and raid the minibar?

And like my client's predicament, this is a time when you really don't have the patience for a lecture or the time to read a tome that will help you understand the psychology of why you overeat or that will educate you on the complex workings of the human digestive system! Nope. It's a whole lot more simple than that: it's one of those times when you just want to look awesome.

No need for an apology at this point. Nothing to be ashamed of. You. Just. Want. To. Look. Awesome.

But how do you—like my celebrity clients—get there? What was my plan for my rock star? And what will I offer you? A Jumpstart. A get-started-right-now with no-more-excuses, three-week plan. You need a kick in the pants, and I'm good at that.

Maybe you are already doing my Skinny Rules and have been losing weight and feeling great . . . but you still want to kick it up a notch for that big event you've got coming up. You too need a kick in the pants and, as I said: I'm good at that!

*Jumpstart to Skinny* is the same exclusive, star-turn regimen that I offered my celebrity friend. In just three weeks, I will get you ready for that special event—and then you can transition to (or go back to) a sustainable regimen (aka *The Skinny Rules*) for the many happy days and years to follow.

In other words, I'm going to Jumpstart you into looking your absolute best!

## MORE MOTIVATION

I'm a fitness expert *and* a self-proclaimed fashion expert, so I do know a thing or two about motivation, and I know how much fashion plays a part.

If you've bought *Jumpstart to Skinny* to get aisle-ready for your wedding or photo-ready for your reunion, you've likely thought a lot about your outfit(s). Yes, that white dress. Or that form-fitting wonder for the class gathering. It probably cost you a pretty penny, and you'd like it to look perfect.

If you've bought *Jumpstart to Skinny* to get beach-ready for your vacation, you've thought a lot about your swimsuit. Yes, that swimsuit. Whether a bikini or a one-piece, Speedo or trunks, there's not a lot of fabric. It's going to show some skin.

Well, whatever the outfit, have you bought it yet? If not, do it. Do it now. Having that outfit or bathing suit hanging in your closet will focus you, will keep your eyes on the prize for the next three weeks.

If you have already bought it, try it on as soon as possible in front of a tough-minded friend and ask for her unvarnished opinion. If it already looks perfect, you're not reading this book! If the verdict is that you could stand to lose a little to look your best, my hunch is that the honest truth will help you stick to my regimen.

When you finish this three-week program, that certain something—your chosen fashion statement—is not only going to fit, it's even going to be comfortable. And you are going to blow people away when they see you in it!

## BUT, BUT . . .

As you might surmise if you've skimmed ahead, you're going to be eating a lot less in the next three weeks than you are used to (which is part of the reason you need my help!).

Like any smart, aware person contemplating a low-calorie diet, you've got some concerns, right?

Before I address them, let me assure you: I am not going to take you anywhere unsafe. Demanding? Yes—you're training with me now, so you know you're not going to get off easy. But unsafe? No.

Trust me, and listen:

*You ask:* But Bob, doesn't such a low-calorie diet go against what you've always said about the importance of a sustainable regimen, and the importance of balance?

*I answer:* Yes, but *you've* decided that you need something special, something fast, and something simple for a *specific date*. And something *short term*. That's the key phrase—this is a short-term change, not a plan you should sustain past your goal date three weeks from now.

So every time you tell me, "But Bob, I can't do this forever," or "But Bob, didn't you say always eat a healthy between-meal snack?" I want you to remember: this is temporary but critical. It is not a permanent regimen, but it *is* one you can break out anytime you need to look your absolute best.

*You ask:* Isn't this going to launch me onto that unhealthy cycle known as yo-yo dieting?

*I answer:* An emerging body of work might reassure you: when scholars at Laval and Sherbrooke Universities compared the after-diet effects of a fifteen-week continuous diet (CD) versus an intermittent diet (ID) of five weeks, they found that "the ID resulted in similar short- *and long-term changes* in body composition and metabolic profile compared with a CD. Most improvements occurred during the first five weeks of treatment in both interventions" (italics mine).

I'm not saying that short-term changes are better than long-term ones; I'm saying . . . don't worry so much, Grandma! And if you transition from the Jumpstart program into my sustainable, long-term regimen—detailed in *The Skinny Rules*—you will enjoy the benefits of both.

*You ask:* Everyone's doing a cleanse diet. Wouldn't that get me where I want to be? Why don't you recommend it?

*I say (kind of sarcastically):* I know, right? Cleanses are cool. They're hip; trendy. And all the celebs are doing them.

Actually, the smarter stars I know *aren't* "cleansing." And there's one very good reason for that: a cleanse—whether a juice fast or a hot water and raw veggie routine—is just too restrictive. Remember: I want you to *complete* this program. I don't want you to get a three-week headache! And I really don't want you to get that heinous bad breath that comes with fasting. Oh, no—not that!

*You persist:* But Bob, I want to do a cleanse because I hear it will literally cleanse my liver! It'll make me feel so much better!

*I ask:* Who have you been talking to? The principal medical societies specializing in liver disease do not recommend cleansing.

The liver, with its highly specialized system of ducts and storage cells, simply *does not work that way*! It must have continuous, high-powered fuel to do its job. Cleansing diets—often just a fast with juice and a high-priced herbal supplement—don't supply that.

As I always say: you've got to eat if you're going to lose weight. It's paradoxical, but it's true. So no cleanse! (But *do* bathe . . .)

*You ask:* Everyone knows you can't lose weight in specific body regions, but that's what I really need to do. I've got some real trouble spots: "bat wings," "muffin tops," back cleavage, and all the rest! There's *no way* I'm waving to my guests before I get in the limo! What can you really do for me, Bob?

*I answer:* While it is true that you can't do exercises that cause regional weight loss, you *can* build up specific muscle groups so that *when you lose weight* those muscles stand out and look great. Interestingly, a recent study of female military personnel showed that women lose arm fat easier than they lose gut and thigh fat—illustrating, once again, that what seems an established fact in nutritional science is always subject to revision. We'll see. . . . The exercises I'm going to give you will, *with the weight loss,* make your body look great. But remember: I have set them up to work *in tandem* with the diet modifications. You've got to do both. Then you can wave bye-bye with pride!

## WHAT TO EXPECT

Here's the breakdown on what's to come.

PART I Here you'll find my Jumpstart Rules. A lucky thirteen. Thirteen things you need to remember (not so hard!) and need to live by for the next three weeks. That's it. Three measly weeks.

You're basically in training for your big event, right? So, think of the Jumpstart Rules as the big reveal version of the final training regimens that athletes (or, in some cases, rock guitarists) use to get ready for *their* big event.

**PART II** Here's where I give you your Jumpstart Day-by-Day Regimen—simple, straightforward food and exercise schedules designed to keep you bright, upbeat, and in command of your body.

**PART III** Next you'll learn my Jumpstart Moves. In Rule 7 you'll learn about my philosophy on strength and toning exercise for this program. For the moment, what you need to know is that you'll be doing one of my seven Jumpstart Move "packages," and the exercises for each routine are demonstrated here.

**PART IV** Get ready for my delicious Jumpstart recipes. Here you'll find twenty-one days of food ideas—power breakfasts, lean lunches, and thinner dinners—designed to meet your Jumpstart calorie and nutrient needs.

## LET ME HEAR YOU SAY IT . . .

*Jumpstart to Skinny* is a pretty demanding but very doable program. If you stick to it, you won't be worrying about flabby arms, unfashionable back cleavage, or even those unsightly bat wings. You will: Just. Look. Totally. Awesome.

So, what happened to my rock star client?

Three weeks after coming to me in a panic, she performed on stage and was hot, hot, hot! She came out often from behind that guitar, I'm telling you. And from the stage she yelled out: "I love you, Bobby!"

So, are you in?

I'd better hear it loud and clear: HELL YES!

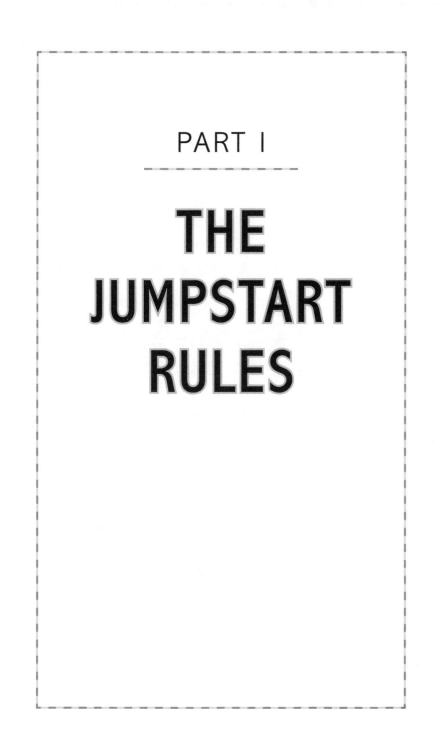

# PART I

# THE JUMPSTART RULES

# RULE 1

## TAKE CONTROL WITH PROPER PROPORTIONS—40/40/20

t's one thing to hand someone a tough battle plan and tell her to "just get going."

It's another to give her the tools to execute said plan and *win the battle.*

I want you to win.

That's what this rule is about.

The 40/40/20 plan is the nutritional architecture of your Jumpstart eating regimen. And it is easy, especially since I've done all the work for you in my menus and recipes!

The 40/40/20 plan is my way of making sure you get the right amount of the three essential macronutrients in your diet: protein, carbohydrates, and fat. Without them, you'd be in trouble. Without them in the right amounts, you'll stay fat, and you'll never get into that dress, tux, Speedo, or bikini. (Of course, you also need fiber, which is why I give you license to eat unlimited quantities of Jumpstart veggies.)

I've tinkered with this formula to get it right: I've tried different percentages, added, subtracted, split things up one week and then tried something new the next. In other words, I have been your guinea pig, and I know this is the formula that will work. Don't make my effort for nothing—use what I've learned!

But I'll back up a step and give you a macronutrient primer:

Protein is a dieter's best friend. Not only does it help maintain muscle while you are losing fat, it can also prevent you from feeling hungry. Why? Because protein helps control blood sugar and insulin—two elements that, out of balance, can make you feel famished and craving all the wrong things. During your Jumpstart program, 40 percent of your calories will come from protein.

Carbohydrates—nature's sugars—are the body's fuel. We need them to keep our energy levels up, to keep our thinking sharp, and to replenish starved muscles. But carbohydrates come in two different forms: simple and complex. I'm oversimplifying, but think of it this way: simple carbohydrates are found in fruits and vegetables (which, again, also give us needed fiber) and are, generally, "good." Complex carbohydrates are what we find in processed starchy food—breads, baked goods, pastas, crackers, and potatoes. It's not that complex carbohydrates are evil or that you can never have them again (you can!), but most people rely too heavily on carbohydrates of the complex variety, and don't get enough simple ones! When we overload on the complex carbs, we wreak havoc on our systems.

If we can control our carb intake—if we *use* them rather than *abuse* them—we can push our body during exercise, and the carbs we have eaten will replenish our starved muscles. As with protein, you're going to be eating 40 percent mostly simple carbohydrates (see Rule 3 about when you can have some complex ones) for the next three weeks.

**NET CARBS**

In addition to simple carbs and complex carbs, there's one more vocabulary word I need to explain here, folks: *net carbs*. Net carbs refers to the amount of carbohydrates in the food after you have considered the way in which the fiber in that food offsets the carb number. A food like, say, blueberries, has 21 grams of carbs per cup, but 4 grams of fiber. So, to calculate the net carbs for a cup of blueberries, you subtract the grams of fiber from the carbs: that's 17 net carbs! You'll see in Part IV that I list the nutritional value of each recipe. When I list the carbs per serving, I'm talking about net carbs.

We also need fats—whether in the form of oils or solids. Fats help maintain the essential barriers around our cells, help keep our skin and various other tissues flexible, and provide a dense source of fuel—120 calories for every tablespoon! Fats are not "bad"—we just need to use the right ones the right way. If we do, we can reduce feelings of hunger and stay on the path to successful weight loss and an awesome big reveal body. Your Jumpstart diet will allow 20 percent fats.

In the daily menus in Part II ("The Jumpstart Day-by-Day Regimen"), I've already calculated your macronutrient diet as close to 40 percent protein, 40 percent carbs, and 20 percent fat as possible for each meal. (Remember that because the fiber in fruits and veggies brings their net carb number down, you may sometimes be getting far fewer than 40 percent carbs from my recipes. But I'm assuming you'll be snacking on fruits and veggies all day long, so you'll get your needed carbs over the course of the day.) Meaning: these proportions are already basically figured into each meal. All you have to do is fix the meal and eat it. No excuses.

So, this is easy math, right? Made easier because I've done the menu planning for you. These proportions—40/40/20—are the same ones I use when *I'm* getting ready for a cover shoot. These are the proportions my celebrity clients use to get red-carpet ready. And they're the proportions *you're* going to use for your own cover shoot. You'll have an amazing, for-the-ages wedding album, a jealousy-inducing reunion photo, a bathing-beauty shot that your spouse just can't stop looking at!

---

### SCREW THE MATH

Last time I checked, 40 plus 40 plus 20 equals 100. And 100 percent of anything is all there is, right? But wait! There's some good news here: I'm going to give you some free calories above and beyond your 40/40/20 allotment. See page 37 for a list of Bob-approved Jumpstart veggies. You'll see in Part II that you'll have many of these vegetables daily, but feel free to add as many you want—more than I have called for!—to your meals. In fact, you'd be crazy not to. These are freebie calories—no need to think about your 40/40/20 proportion when you are eating them.

In addition to possibly satisfying your urge to just munch on something, these veggies will ensure you are getting lots of fiber. And more of the *right kind* of fiber means greater—and healthier—weight loss.

---

# RULE 2

-------------

## CUT BACK ON CALORIES. THEN CUT BACK AGAIN.

B race yourself for the truth: for this diet to work on time (three weeks!), you should eat 800 calories a day if you're female and 1,200 calories a day if you're male.

Why did I say brace yourself? Most diet experts and motivators prefer to keep people in the dark about calorie restriction, but they all know the truth. They dress it up in pretty prose but never tell you the truth about the number of calories it takes (or doesn't take) to meet your goals. I think you deserve my honesty. You're an adult: you can take the truth in plain terms.

Are you miffed at me for being so hard on you? That's OK. I can take it. Remember: I spend most of my time convincing ravenously hungry obese people *not* to eat! And, believe me, they've said some choice things to me about that.

But here's what they usually say about it later: thanks, Bob, I needed that!

They, like you, *get* it: special circumstances call for aggressive measures. *Jumpstart to Skinny* is not a permanent regimen. But it is safe, and it will get you into that dress, Speedo, or bikini.

And that, if I remember right, is what this is all about for you. Keep your eyes on the prize.

Now, where do those numbers—800 for women, 1,200 for men—come from? In short, they come from years of experience with clients in your shoes. They come from years of my *trying* to be accommodating, sensitive, and empathetic when folks said things like, "Can't you just give me a little more food?" or "Bob, can't you let me have a tablespoon of peanut butter or something before bed? After all, protein is good for weight loss. Right, Bob?"

Yes, I tried to be compassionate, I tried to be Mr. Sympathy— and my clients didn't meet their weight-loss goals.

There is just no way around it. You've got to ratchet your intake way down if you want a skinnier you.

All that said, it's not just calories in, calories out that makes for weight loss. It's also what's *in* those calories that counts. That's why—as you'll see—I'm so specific about what you should eat and when you should eat it. The 800/1,200 model works. Trust my process, OK?

Or you could trust the science:

What you'll be embarking on for the next three weeks is known as a very low-calorie diet, or VLCD in nutritionist terms. One conventional whack against very low-calorie diets concerns weight *re*gain—what happens when you go off the aggressive regimen. A nation of diet relapsers tells us there's no doubt that regain happens. We are not entirely sure why. But we do now know that regain is not an inevitable outcome of VLCDs.

As early as 1995, researchers at the University of Pittsburgh School of Medicine concluded that "just 7 days of caloric restriction can produce dramatic improvements in glycemic control;

moreover, *VLCDs produce greater improvements in glycemic control than more moderate diets, even if weight losses are the same.*" With my added emphasis in italics, that means that better glycemic control means better weight control.

More recently, a giant and ongoing study in the European Union has been trying to connect the dots between success in losing weight and success in maintaining that loss. One of its interim findings, just published as I was writing this, concludes that "LCD (low calorie diet)-induced changes in BMI [and] fasting insulin . . . are inversely associated with weight regain in the 6-month period following weight loss." In other words: the positive metabolic changes that the low-calorie diet induced made weight regain much less likely.

And another study, from Maastricht University in the Netherlands: "VLCD *with active follow-up treatment* seems to be one of the better treatment modalities related to long-term weight-maintenance success" (italics mine).

In other words, short-term very low-calorie dieting *can* produce a whole bunch of positive changes that will keep you from getting fat again. The trial is not over, and the jury is certainly not out. It's still hearing evidence. But, again, the more I observe my own clients and the more I study, the more convinced I've become: in the short run, it's the way to go. And right this moment, you're in the short run. Eight hundred calories for women. Twelve hundred for men. Got it?

All of which means: at nine o'clock at night, when you're dreaming about food and ruminating over this Jumpstart Rule, you'll hate my guts!

But trust me: when you're walking down the aisle, you'll want to kiss me.

Oh yes, brothers and sisters, you will!

# RULE 3

---

# EAT NO COMPLEX CARBS
# AFTER BREAKFAST

When you transition to my Skinny Rules for your permanent way of eating, you'll see that I would like you to keep your complex carb munching to the morning and midday hours. That is, no bread or pasta or crackers or potatoes after lunch. That is a great long-term way to eat. In normal circumstances, I wouldn't monkey with it.

But these are not normal circumstances.

This is a campaign—leading to a final, memorable victory lap.

And for that, we need to ratchet everything up. Hence: we're going to limit complex carbohydrate consumption to breakfast. Lunch and dinner we're going lean and green!

Recall the basics. Complex carbs (even whole grains) are forms of sugar, and sugar cues the pancreas to make more insulin. And that process triggers appetite! Simple carbohydrates—like the kind found in fruits and veggies—don't react in the body the same way, partly because the fiber in fruits and vegetables offsets the carb load. This is why I am OK with you eating as many veggies throughout the day as you like, but I want you to eat fruit only as I've prescribed in my menus (and, as you'll find out in Rule 11, you'll be knocking off fruits entirely in week 3). But for the next three weeks, you've simply got to lay off the complex ones after your power breakfast!

Why does it matter what time of day you eat carbohydrates? Well, think about that appetite trigger. The later in the day you eat complex carbs, the more likely it is that you will get food cravings late at night. To Jumpstart your weight loss, we're just dialing the clock back a bit.

I didn't rework this rule just to be a hard-ass trainer. I thought a lot about the total package of demands I was making here, and this one made the cut. Why? Basic nutritional science and twenty-five years of training experience: eating fewer complex carbs works. By doing so, you signal your body to burn more fat than it usually would. Not eating complex carbs late in the day works. By doing so, you hold off the cravings I mention above. Simple.

---

**REACH FOR A SIMPLE CARB**

Experience tells me that eliminating starch carbs after breakfast is easier than eliminating simple carbs. For one thing, it's easier to snack on an apple (simple carb) than on a bowl of pasta (a big ole bowl of complex). Two, I find that simple carbs tend to keep my brain—and my thinking!—clearer, whereas complex carbohydrates make me a little sleepy. Stay sharp and focused; you can sleep later!

To make rationing your calories to 800/1,200 tolerable and to make up for the carbs you might like to be eating after breakfast, I've created my menus with a couple of important things in mind. For starters, I've given you protein in all of your meals so you'll feel fuller (and less likely to crave the complex carbs). My menus also combine fat and simple carbs in a way that works well for me and for my clients—again, you'll feel more full and less crabby. And remember, when it comes to the vegetables on my recommended list, you can forget about calories; you'll get virtually unlimited vegetables—fiber!—all day long.

## THE BEST SIMPLE CARBS FOR THE BEST BODY

Fruits are simple carbohydrates. When in doubt, I prefer high-fiber fruits since they tend to be lower in net carbs, because they have more . . . fiber! The latter aids weight loss in two ways. One, the obvious: it helps *move things along* faster. Two, the fiber slows down and offsets the sugar surge from the fruit's natural sugar. That's why we call them *net* carbs. But they *are* sugars, so I've parceled them out in your daily regimens—as part of your 40/40/20 calorie budget. Here are a few fruits that I eat all the time:

apples
blueberries
blackberries
kiwi
strawberries

# RULE 4

------------

## GET RID OF WATER WEIGHT BY DRINKING MORE WATER

'm a little, eh, *intense* about water. I know I am. But for good reason. The more I learn about water, and the more I work with contestants on *The Biggest Loser* and with private clients, the more convinced I am of its importance. Let me count the ways. . . .

For starters, drinking water before every meal will make you eat less because the water will make you feel a little full before you eat. That's a no-brainer.

Second, simply staying sufficiently hydrated can increase your resting rate of metabolism, or resting energy expenditure (REE). That means that just by drinking water your body will burn more calories than if you were underhydrated or dehydrated. When you look at it that way, there's really no excuse not to drink water all the time.

Next, there's the scientifically complex but pretty straightforward truth that increased water intake lets the liver devote more resources to fat metabolism—which is what we want, right?

But now things start to get a little strange: drinking *more* water leads to retaining *less* water, and, hence, losing water weight.

I always wondered about this during my early years spent in some of LA's most aggressive body-building gyms. There, the fittest, toughest, most dedicated women and men were *not* carrying around nice little one-pint bottles of water. They were carrying one-gallon *jugs* of water! They all had the same explanation: "You can't lose the water weight without drinking a lot of water, Bob!"

Here's the short course on what's really going on: drinking lots of water "tricks" the body into shedding water more efficiently. Just as the body starts storing fat when confronted with a food fast (shifting into its starvation/survival mode), so too does the body store water when confronted with water deprivation. In a strange way, by changing your water drinking habits you also shift the way your body deals with water—you "train it to shed it" instead of holding on to it.

Your ankles will love you forever!

All of this is pretty cool to know, sure, but of the other supportive studies on water, guess which study interests me the most? Is it the one about how hydration improves cardiovascular outcomes? The one about water and your skin?

Or could it possibly be this one? "Water Consumption Increases Weight Loss During a Hypocaloric Diet Intervention"?

Clear skin is a nice byproduct, but I think you know which study is most relevant here!

Let's check in on it . . .

In 2010, a group of researchers for the Institute for Public Health and Water Research decided to further explore the water–weight loss connection. They already knew what we know: that pre-meal water consumption "acutely reduces energy intake" or, in plain English, makes you eat less because you feel full. Now they wanted to know something else: does it *lead to actual weight loss*, and is that weight loss temporary or sustainable? To find out, they divided a group of forty-eight chubby adults into two groups. Half of the group ate their low-calorie meals after drinking 500 milliliters of water (a little more than 16 ounces); the other group ate the same low-calorie meals, but without the water. Twelve weeks later they were weighed.

Results? Not only did the water drinkers lose four more pounds than the nondrinkers, they also tended to sustain that weight loss over time. The story just gets more and more interesting. Conclusion? "When combined with a hypocaloric diet, consuming 500 ml water prior to each main meal leads to greater weight loss than a hypocaloric diet alone . . . This may be due in part to an acute reduction in meal EI [energy intake] following water ingestion."

I'll take it!

## JUMPSTART AMOUNTS OF $H_2O$

My recommendation in *The Skinny Rules* was to drink 16 ounces (two large glasses) of water before every meal and every snack, or a total of 80 ounces over the course of the day. To Jumpstart your weight loss, that's the *minimum* amount I want you to be throwing back every day. I won't lie to you: this will require some thought and planning on your part because you won't be snacking for the next three weeks, and so will get an automatic prompt to drink 16 ounces only three times a day instead of five (three meals and two snacks—five prompts!). But this isn't that hard, people. For one thing, if you follow the day-by-day regimen (Part II), you will be drinking enough before and during each meal and activity. But if you don't drink as much as is prescribed there, you can keep up the pace of water intake by following some of the tips in the box below ("Make Your Own Water Reminders").

There is, of course, a price for all this guzzling, and I think you know what it is. You'll pee like a racehorse. But don't worry! Peeing just means you're shedding water weight. And that's why you're drinking so much of it, right?

---

**MAKE YOUR OWN WATER REMINDERS**

Is it possible to make yourself more water-conscious during the run-up to your big reveal? It is. Set yourself up for success:

- Keep full bottles in your car, and keep one in the cup holder at all times.
- Put a large glass or bottle next to the kitchen sink as well as one next to your bed.
- Put a bottle of water in your bottom desk drawer (every time you open the drawer—surprise!—it's water time), and keep one on your desktop at all times.
- Keep a bottle of lemon or lime juice visible—it will remind you that you can change the taste of water when you are bored with . . . water.
- Buy inexpensive, no-sugar, flavored club soda and make infused no-cal "mocktails" at night.

# RULE 5

-- -- -- -- -- -- --

## GET YOUR ELECTROLYTES

Because this regimen demands a little more sweat than you may be used to, it requires a little more attention to nutritional basics. I'm going to make sure that you properly supplement your normal intake of electrolytes so you recover faster from exercise and stay energized.

Electrolytes are minerals—sodium, potassium, magnesium, calcium, chloride, hydrogen phosphate, and hydrogen carbonate. You don't need to memorize that list, but you *do* need to be sure you get enough of them. Especially during the Jumpstart, when you are pushing your body with exercise and limiting your calories.

Electrolytes help maintain the fluid balance inside and outside your cells. Muscle contraction—the essence of muscle building—becomes impossible when you don't get enough electrolytes. Muscles weaken, and you get cramps. Not fun. If your electrolyte count is severely disturbed, you get cardiac and neurological problems, and you can wind up in the emergency ward. Really not fun. Especially before your reunion, wedding, or vacation!

---

**ELECTROLYTES THE OLD-FASHIONED WAY**

Where do electrolytes hide in your food? Fruit and veggies, people!
Chomp away:

For potassium: lemons, strawberries, blueberries, blackberries

For sodium: bell peppers, leaf lettuce, celery, radishes

For magnesium: spinach and radishes

For calcium: broccoli, celery, onions, apples

---

So how, exactly, can you make sure you're getting the critical minerals and vitamins you need to stay bright-eyed and bushy-tailed during your Jumpstart regimen? It's not that hard.

You can get these minerals from your diet, and if you weren't working out five times a week with me, that would probably be enough. But you will be working out five times a week, won't you? Therefore, you'll need to supplement. You'll see in my daily guidelines that you'll be drinking 8 ounces of electrolyte replacement twice a day. You have two options:

1. After decades of irresponsibly selling high-sugar electrolyte replacements in the form of "sports drinks," manufacturers finally get it: we don't want or need the sugar. We just need the electrolytes, thank you. If you plan to replenish your electrolytes this way, be sure to read the drink labels! If a drink has any sweeteners—natural or artificial—leave it there on the shelf or in the fridge. Buy the one with minimum additives and maximum minerals and vitamins.

2. You can also get your dose via the many powdered electrolyte replacements now on the market, which means, as a practical

matter, that you'll be killing two birds with one stone (getting your electrolytes *and* some of the water you need). Just add the powder to the water you need to be drinking anyway and you're on your way. I use a brand called Electro-Mix. I like it because I can adjust the amount I want for any given amount of water. It is also cheaper than many other brands. Money matters when you're getting ready for a pricey vacation.

---

**TAKE *NO* LAXATIVES OR DIURETICS. PERIOD.**

When it comes to diets, believe me, I've seen it all: Magic herbs and fruits. Secret workouts. Outright idiocy, let's face it. Yet there *is* one common dieting practice that outright scares me—sends me yelling, "Don't do it!"

What is it?

Laxatives.

I understand why you'd consider using them. But do you really want to (1) feel like hell all the time, (2) look haggard and washed out, (3) spend all your time on the can reading five-year-old *People* magazines, and (4) kinda have to . . . *run* down the aisle at your wedding?

How about having to sprint over everyone else on the beach while you—sweating, panicky, flushed, and crazy—seek one of those funky beach bathrooms?

I thought you'd say that.

If you need a reminder of these things, let me give you a list of the worst laxative effects:

Intestinal injury
Abdominal pain, bloating, and fullness
Dehydration

Electrolyte abnormalities

Really irritable bowel syndrome

Ulceration of the bowel

Exacerbation of hemorrhoids

Esophagitis

Gastritis

Gastric ulceration

Gastric bleeding

Intestinal injury

Esophageal perforations and lacerations

Malabsorption of nutrients leading to hypoproteinemia, hypoalbumin-
emia, and calcium deficiency

Fatty infiltration of the liver

Pancreatitis

Still interested in taking laxatives? I didn't think so.

Now you ask: What about prescription "water pills" or so-called natural diuretics? My clear answer: unless they are prescribed for high blood
pressure, no.

Come on! Have you been listening to Captain Bob? Remember:
we're using water, diet (veggies, high-fiber fruits!), and exercise to do
all of this without messing you up! Trust me. Throw out the pills. If I find
out you're using them, I'll lock the bathroom door on you, soldier!

# RULE 6

## DO 45 MINUTES A DAY OF LOW-INTENSITY CARDIO, PREFERABLY BEFORE BREAKFAST

Yes, cardio every day. And I'll get to the "preferably before breakfast" clause in a minute. This might sound rather demanding. But the kind of cardio I'm calling for here is low intensity, so don't freak out. Low-intensity work stretches out your muscles, revs up your metabolism, and gets you psyched for the day. No one is asking you to get to the gym for jazz aerobics before breakfast! Low intensity—relax.

Need more encouragement? Think about three weeks from now: Will you be happy about jogging along the beach or walking down the aisle, or will your arms be flapping in the wind? You obviously want the former—and so do I. You are going to look amazing *and* healthy when I'm done with you!

If you're still feeling highly tense about my low-intensity rule, put my picture on a dartboard and have at it. (Note to self: explore potential of dart-throwing as triceps exercise.)

So, how much? While you are on the Jumpstart program, I want you to put in 45 minutes of low-intensity exercise every day. I suggest walking. It's simple; you can do it alone, with a friend, or with your dog; and you don't need any equipment. Walking—that's the ticket! The key, I want to emphasize again, is low intensity. If you can't talk easily while doing it, slow down. If you feel like going to sleep, go faster!

But I know what you're thinking: what's with . . . the *last three words* in that rule?

*Preferably before breakfast?* You *must* be kidding, Bob. At the very least, you ask: Is it worth the pain?

In short, yes. In my work with clients and contestants, I've seen the pattern: those who exercise before eating tend to (a) stay on the diet and (b) lose more weight.

There is a significant psychological factor at play here, and I think you know what I'm talking about: the longer a person frets, postpones, and rationalizes away his daily exercise commitment, the more likely he is to, let us say, forget it altogether—or at least spend the day justifying why today, well, it's OK to "take a break." Get your exercise out of the way *first thing* in the morning and you won't have to think about when you'll make time for it. And when you exercise every day, you will lose weight.

But there is also some emerging science on exercise metabolics—how your body handles challenge and change. It suggests that exercise on an empty stomach has a direct link to weight loss in and of itself.

Here's what we know so far: when you exercise in a fasted or semifasted state (which is more or less what you are when you haven't yet eaten breakfast), you are drawing on body reserves of fat and carbohydrates. That is what we want, right? I admit that some science also suggests that eating before exercise might be better for daylong fat burning. But the problem with that suggestion is that it hasn't yet been determined *how much* or exactly *what* you should eat to get that daylong fat-burning benefit. Besides, still other research shows something else: you clearly burn more fat *during* exercise when you do it in a fasted state.

A couple of details bear mention:

University of Birmingham researchers studying exercise physiology recently collected and analyzed a large number of studies on fat oxidation rates in various states: fasting, semifasting, and fed. (Fat oxidation: good.) They also varied the intensity of exercise training required to induce changes in fat oxidation. (Again: what we want!) Their findings: "Ingestion of carbohydrate in the hours before or on commencement of exercise reduces the rate of fat oxidation significantly compared with fasted conditions, whereas fasting longer than 6 h[ours] optimizes fat oxidation."

So, the jury might still be out in terms of a binding verdict, but I read these studies as encouraging proof of what I see in my work with clients and contestants: exercising on an empty stomach works.

---

### I CAN'T FUNCTION WITHOUT MY CAFFEINE

Many people resist doing anything in the morning before they've had some caffeine. If that describes you, good news here! I am all for letting you get your caffeine fix in the morning, so long as you don't add milk, cream, or artificial sweetener (or more than a very little bit of real sugar). See Rule 13 for more about why you should be drinking espresso!

**COMMON SENSE FOR EARLY-MORNING EXERCISE**

If I didn't tell you that occasionally a client feels weak or dizzy upon undertaking this tough step, I'd be lying. But I've got a few suggestions that will help you out if this proves to be a problem:

1. If you get dizzy, bring yourself slowly to your knees, then lean over, as if you were (a) resting in yoga, (b) praying, or (c) doing the "I'm not worthy" thing from the movie *Wayne's World*. This is the classic, nearly instinctive way of dealing with any kind of dizziness, whether caused by things like antidepressants, blood pressure meds, or certain preexisting conditions. Then slowly come back up to kneeling, then standing. Try the exercise again, slowly—don't give up entirely. If you are still woozy, you know what to do: sit it out, eat breakfast, and try again tomorrow.

2. Look at your face in the mirror. If you've been following my regimen, you should look good—maybe a little flushed, but good. If you look haggard or pale, sit down, put your head between your knees for a few minutes, then hydrate with an electrolyte replacement.

3. Next time, get a friend to work out with you. Remember: prebreakfast exercise is moderate. Save your more intense work for later in the day, when you're fueled up.

4. Keep drinking water and your electrolyte replacement—before, during, and after exercise.

5. If you repeatedly feel nauseous, dizzy, or generally awful when exercising in a fasted state, then by all means eat first. But do the cardio at some point every day (try the walk at lunchtime instead, if you can, or before dinner) or be prepared to look chubby in three weeks.

# RULE 7

---

# FIVE TIMES A WEEK, AT ANY TIME OF DAY, DO 15 TO 20 MINUTES OF MY JUMPSTART MOVES

D id you think that walking or other low-intensity morning exercise was all you'd need to do for the next three weeks to be ready for your big day or event?

Think again!

No apologies here: this program works. But you have to do the whole thing. So, find fifteen to twenty minutes, five times a week. That's not a lot of time, people. You can do this! You can make the time.

In Part III, I'll show you exactly how to execute my exercises and in what combination. For now, however, I just want to introduce you to the concept, the philosophy behind my moves. It's all about metabolic conditioning, or met-con for short.

Met-con works the whole body quickly, efficiently. Met-con movements use your own body weight to slim and trim yourself for the long, lean look you desire. All you need are a little space in your house (or office or hotel!), medium hand weights or a kettle-bell, a jump rope, a medicine ball, and an exercise band (though if you don't have one of the last two, you can substitute another exercise routine on that day). If you want to ramp up the intensity, you can do some advanced movements that use a medicine ball. With met-con movements, you will be flexing, stretching, and streamlining your whole body.

Take, for example, the "burpee," which is one of the met-con exercises you'll do as part of your fifteen- to twenty-minute program, five times a week. (I'm repeating that because I want you to focus on how little the time investment really is! You can do this!)

The burpee, also known as the squat thrust, gives the benefits of both strength training and aerobic work. Its origins and importance are telling. It was created by an American physiologist named Royal H. Burpee for the purpose of evaluating overall physical fitness. Later on, the army used the move to measure the battle readiness of new recruits during World War II. A generation of soldiers brought it into civilian life, where its fortunes waxed and waned over the next fifty years.

I think it should be hot all the time!

Let me walk you through a burpee and explain what's going on when you do it.

You start out standing, then drop into a squat position and place your hands on the ground. In one quick move, extend your feet back to the classic plank position (like at the beginning of a push-up). From here you drop your chest and hips onto the floor and then in one motion, return to the squat position, and jump straight up into the air.

OK, quick and without overthinking: What, exactly, is happening to your body while doing the burpee? For one thing, by alternating and changing up exercise movements, you help delay a phenomenon in the science of movement known as adaptation— your muscles don't get a chance to "figure out" how to minimize caloric expenditure. Second, in the burpee, you can *feel* your whole body stretching, flexing, and contracting while your heart pumps faster and harder. You're working those big muscle groups that tend to burn more calories.

In Part III, you'll take up a number of these met-con moves. I'll give them to you in seven distinct "packages" or specific routines at the bottom of each day's calendar. You'll see that I've suggested which met-con package you should do each day, but you choose the one you want to do, so long as you do a different one on each of your five exercise days. Most of the packages don't require anything more than a hand weight or kettlebell and a jump rope, but don't let me hear you excusing yourself because you don't have a weight or a rope. No weight? Use something else that's heavy enough to make you sweat. No rope? Pretend you have one and go through the motions!

I encourage you to write down the number of reps you were able to do easily, how many in total, and how long the entire package took you. You'll be surprised to see your progress if you review these notes as you go.

Know this for sure: you will never be bored with these met-con routines. And, as you likely know, nothing kills a good fitness regimen faster than boredom.

You are not going to be bored. Promise.

## CROSSFIT?

In the world I inhabit, trendy workout routines come and go as fast as flatulence after a burrito! It seems like there's always a new exercise fad: from Pilates to Zumba to hot yoga to whatever else is hot at the moment. In my opinion, the best workout out there is CrossFit. I'm a big fan and go to CrossFit "boxes" (really just CrossFit workout spaces) wherever I can find them, even when I'm traveling.

CrossFit may be popular, but it's not a pop-up fad set to the latest music or exercise gadget. The whole culture is about strength and conditioning through hard work, and the routines are, get this, made up mostly of met-con movements! Which is to say, classic stretching and conditioning movements.

But understand this: you don't have to go to a box! You can do this at home. You're not going to do any strength or conditioning moves anywhere near as intense as you'd do in a CrossFit box!

You are, however, going to love what you see in the mirror in three weeks!

# RULE 8

---

## CUT THE SALT

Aren't you reading this book because you're in need of a fast-acting weight-loss program? Then don't give me any attitude about this rule being a giant "duh!" I know you've probably heard that too much salt is bad, and you've likely also heard that we all eat too much of it. But my guess is that you don't have a clear sense of how much is too much and how much you consume.

If you eat packaged or processed foods (which I really wish you wouldn't!), you're probably already getting more salt than you need. Even if you are careful to buy and eat "low-sodium" packaged or processed foods, think again—unless you eat the tiny "serving size," you are shoveling in the salt. I mean, really, twelve low-salt potato chips equals a serving?

Yes, your body needs some salt to stay in chemical balance (which is why you'll be drinking electrolyte replacements during this program), but too much leads to water retention, which leads nowhere good. If you haven't been doing so already, it's past high time you started paying close attention to your salt intake!

The standard advice if you're not trying to lose weight is to consume *no more* than 2,300 milligrams of salt a day. I aim lower— when you're looking to lose weight over the long haul and then stay thin, you should shoot for less than 2,000 milligrams a day.

But now that you're trying to Jumpstart your weight loss, I'm asking you to cut your salt again. For the next three weeks, you're aiming for 1,000 milligrams a day. That keeps you within the safety zone of the FDA's daily minimum requirement while further reducing your water-retaining sodium.

Don't freak out: 500 milligrams equals one-fifth of a teaspoon. Do they even make measuring spoons in an increment that small? No! You're not going to miss this little bit of salt. If you follow my meal plans and recipes, you won't even have to think about salt and how to get just the right amount. My plan won't let you exceed 1,000 milligrams a day.

If you're not following my meals and recipes but want to cook for yourself, keep these "how to eat less salt" tips in mind:

- Squeeze lemon juice on your food to enhance flavor.
- Cook with more herbs.
- Read food labels carefully, keeping an eye out for serving size and the amount of sodium per serving.
- Use less salt than your recipe calls for. You can always add more if the dish really needs it; you can never take salt out!
- Don't have a salt shaker on your table—why tempt yourself? (This isn't just a Jumpstart idea—you don't need that shaker on the table, ever.)

## AVOIDING SALT

There likely will be times when you can't stay home and make one of my recipes. In that case, you have to ask about or guess at the amount of salt in a dish . . . and often that means you should pass it by. Consider these situations.

At a friend's house for dinner: Ask ahead what he's serving. He's a friend. Don't be shy. If it's starch-heavy, ask about the protein and the veggie. He's a friend. Impose a little. It's OK.

At dinner at your boss's home: How could he schedule this now? So insensitive! OK, you don't want to be rude here, right? So, pick around the plate, and if you slip, no worries! You'll get back on the horse the next day. Trust me.

On the road: When filling the tank, do not go into the minimart. Take raw string beans and Persian cucumbers with you on the road.

At the airport: Stride quickly past the snack-food joints on both sides of you. Take string beans and Persian cucumbers instead!

At a bar: Girl, are you at a bar? See Rule 12.

At your mother-in-law's house for dinner: Just don't go over there; she can't cook anyway.

At an office party: Stay away from the snack table unless raw veggies are present. Focus on the hot young intern.

# RULE 9

- - - - - - - - -

## TAKE ADVANTAGE OF THE RESTORATIVE POWER OF DAILY FISH OIL

You may have heard that taking a fish oil supplement every day is good for your heart. That may be true, but as scientists have studied fish oil supplementation and chronic illness, they've come across the benefits of fish oil for people who diet and exercise as well. Fish oil can help with post-exercise soreness and also boost immunity.

And you are going to be exercising, right? Your low-intensity morning exercise shouldn't cause next-day soreness, but your met-con workouts probably will. Will you continue to exercise if you are stiff or sore? Maybe. But my experience tells me that you might just use it as an excuse to delay your next workout. I can hear the rationalization now: "I'm a little sore today. I must have done more than was necessary yesterday. I think I can afford to take a day off from met-con this week."

This is a three-week program, people! You can't push off until tomorrow what you must do today. No excuses: do your workouts and take your fish oil.

In August 2012, researchers at China's Zhejiang University published a revealing study about fish oil's anti-inflammatory, anti-soreness role. Bear with me: in the human inflammatory cycle, a molecule dubbed E2, or PGE2 (for prostaglandin), signals other cells to become inflamed and, thus, painful. So the research question was: Can we inhibit this process in a healthy way?

To find out, the investigators tested the effects of eight different dietary oils containing high amounts of the anti-inflammatory molecule called docosahexaenoic acid. Result: "It was identified that fish oil best inhibited the PGE2 signaling . . . [and] docosahexaenoic acid (DHA), found in abundance in fish oil, was identified as a key factor of inhibition of PGE2 signaling."

In essence: yay fish oil!

I've been using it ever since, and the soreness has all but disappeared. As a guy whose business it is to exercise, I'd have to say: it's changed my life.

So sometimes, experimenting for *you* confers great benefits on *me*!

I'll take it, and so should you—and I mean after your big reveal as well!

---

**OTHER SUPPLEMENTS?**

Don't stop taking your multivitamin. A good daily multi is a must; the list on the back of the bottle will tell you if the dose fulfills the recommended daily allowances (RDA), but double-check that it contains at least 1,000 milligrams of calcium and 600 international units (IU) of Vitamin D.

A number of great things happen to your body when you exercise, but when you're combining daily exercise with a very low-calorie diet, you want to make sure your immune system is up to the challenge. New research coming out of the Institute of Medical Science in Aberdeen, Scotland, shows that fish oil can boost the main molecules responsible for the immune response.

Researchers took sixteen male subjects and put them in a six-week trial involving two groups (fish oil or placebo oil, 3 grams/day). Subjects went in for two visits, the first involving a maximal exercise test (in which the participant walks or runs as fast as he can until he must stop) and the second involving a one-hour bout of endurance exercise on a stationary bike at 70 percent effort (the subject can stop, but must resume the exercise until the hour is over). The investigators then measured immune system molecules at various stages of the experiment. Results: fish oil consistently and significantly raised immune-boosting molecules during the recovery phase of exercise.

That's what we want, especially in the run-up to the big day. I don't want you dragging your butt down the aisle!

## SO HOW MUCH FISH OIL SHOULD YOU TAKE?

This is simple: you're looking to get 3,000 milligrams of fish oil into you every day. Most brands package fish oil in increments of 1,000, so the label should read "1,000 mg omega-3 fatty acids." Got that?

Why? Because the science shows that 2,000 milligrams is the minimum dose of fish oil for anti-inflammatory benefits, and 3,000 milligrams or more is the dosage used in the important studies of fish oil and muscle soreness. I happen to take 5,000 milligrams of fish oil a day, but I'm working out all the time. That's my job! Three thousand is my prescription for what you'll be doing these three weeks. You wouldn't change a prescription on the way to the drugstore, would you? Stick with 3,000 milligrams.

That said, you've got some alternatives. You can simply take one 1,000-milligram fish oil gel caplet at each meal (which is the way I've laid it out for you in the day-by-day regimen). Or you can get fish oil in liquid form. Read the label; as with the gelcaps, most brands will tell you how many spoonfuls to take for that 1,000-milligram increment. Multiply times three.

If you are a person who gets queasy taking a lot of supplements, shop around for what is often called "pharmaceutical-grade fish oil," which just means that it's been processed enough to make it more palatable.

# RULE 10

---

## FALL BACK ON VEGGIES!

I f there was ever a perfect time to make vegetables—greens, reds, and yellows—the centerpiece of your daily diet, now is that time. You've got an important goal, a deadline for that goal, and a demanding diet regimen that calls for every trick in the book to keep you on track.

Though I'm a fan of *all* vegetables and would certainly rather have you eating any kind instead of almost all other categories of food, I encourage you to rely most heavily on *greens* during your three-week Jumpstart. You'll find great greens recipes in Part IV, but you can also eat many of them raw—just rinse and start chomping!

Repeat after me: If you're hungry, eat veggies. If you're bored, eat veggies. If you're hungry and bored, eat veggies. Remember, on this diet you can eat *as many of the veggies listed below as you like*, whenever you want, so take advantage of this all-you-can-eat buffet.

Why do I love vegetables so much?

First, they are a great source of all the vitamins and minerals—

from A to Z—you need for optimum health and overall fitness. In a short-term, demanding regimen like this one, getting your essential vitamins and minerals is more important than ever.

Second, all vegetables, and especially green ones, contain tons of fiber, and we all know what that means—better digestion and faster, regular, and more natural bowel movements.

But here's something you might not already know: they act as natural diuretics. The fibers and chemicals in asparagus, for example, have even been studied as serious blood pressure treatments. You are going to eat a lot of asparagus.

---

**MY UNLIMITED JUMPSTART VEGGIES**

All you can eat . . . when's the last time you heard those words as part of a diet? Stock up on the following vegetables. Could they be any easier to prepare? Rinse them and eat them raw. Cut them into fun-to-eat strips. Boil or microwave them if you prefer your veggies hot or softer. Add them to my recipes. No excuses—try these:

| | |
|---|---|
| arugula | chard |
| asparagus | chili peppers |
| beet greens | chives |
| bell peppers (red, yellow, green) | collard greens |
| | cucumbers |
| bok choy | dandelion greens |
| broccoli, Broccoflower, Broccolini, and rapini | eggplant |
| | endive |
| Brussels sprouts | escarole |
| cabbage (green and red) | fennel |
| cauliflower | green beans |
| celery | green onions (scallions) |

---

| | |
|---|---|
| jicama | radicchio |
| kale | radishes |
| kohlrabi | spinach |
| leeks | summer squash |
| lettuce | tomatoes |
| mushrooms | turnip greens |
| mustard greens | watercress |
| okra | zucchini |
| parsley | |

# RULE 11

------------

## NO FRUIT DURING WEEK 3

I f you're familiar with *The Skinny Rules,* you know I'm a firm
believer in eating an apple and some berries every day. Mainly,
this is because these delicious fruits are naturally high in fiber
and low in calories. As I said in Rule 3, fruit is a simple carb, but
ordinarily I'm OK with you eating fruit all day because its fiber fills
you up and keeps you regular. Also, of course, low-calorie snacking
is a no-brainer if you're trying to, er, consume fewer calories.

As you come to the final lap of the Jumpstart program, however, I'm going to modify your approach to fruit because in addition to fiber, it contains fructose, and that's something that needs
a tad more watching as you get close to your big moment.

Fructose sits at the center of a huge health controversy. First, a
primer: fructose is a form of sugar that predominantly comes from
fruits. Its metabolic profile is different from that of sucrose (usually made from cane or beet sugar) in one critical way: overcon-
sumption of it skews our metabolism toward fat storage rather
than fat burning. Many believe that our stepped-up consumption
of fructose, usually through ingestion of all that high-fructose

corn syrup (HFCS) in soft and "fruit" drinks, plays a key factor in America's twin scourges of obesity and diabetes. That's why New York passed its ban on large soft drinks recently. Other researchers, both in and out of the soft drink and fast-food industries, believe that HFCS has been unjustly maligned, pointing out that the syrup contains only 5 to 10 percent more fructose than regular sugar.

I wonder what those guys would say if their mother's prescription for, say, Lipitor, contained 10 percent more than she was supposed to take!

My riff on the whole issue has been: cut your sugars and you cut the culprits. About fructose as a nutrient in and of itself I have not fretted. I've advocated plenty of fruits—apples, berries, and so on—and I've been content to know that any sugars in them—fructose, sucrose, etc.—get slowed down, metabolically speaking, by the fruit's high fiber content. That's my usual riff, and it's held its own.

But these are not usual times. We are on a performance-event schedule, like Ryan Gosling or Channing Tatum getting ready for a bare-chested film, or Madonna prepping for an amazing new tour. (Does the woman *ever* get just plain tired? She does not!) We want every edge we can get!

And you don't have to take my word for it. Again, there's some science we need to consider. In a nutshell, investigators at University Hospital Zurich wondered this: we know that there is ample data showing adverse health effects from *high* consumption of processed fruit sugars—from insulin resistance to rapid weight gain. But what about *average* consumption by guys who, generally, watch their diet?

The researchers divided subjects into two groups of healthy, normal-weight male volunteers (age 21–25). They all had to consume four different sweetened beverages for three weeks each:

medium fructose at 40 grams/day, then high fructose, high glucose, and high sucrose, each at 80 grams/day.

After measuring the insulin, fat, and in-body glucose response to each drink regimen, they found a surprise: the liver—the organ responsible for regulating the production of blood sugar and insulin—underperformed on the high and medium fructose drinks.

Translation: it did not do a good job of driving down blood glucose, and, more importantly, it impaired insulin sensitivity. What do we know about impaired insulin sensitivity? Yes, it leads to type 2 diabetes.

But what, you ask, does it have to do (at least right now) with *my* priority—looking great in that bathing suit? Simple: impaired insulin sensitivity makes it tougher to lose weight!

So, though you are allowed fruit for two-thirds of the Jumpstart plan, you need to live without it for the last week. Does one week of this really make a difference? Yes. It's one more way to cut calories, one more way to push your body into fat-burning mode, one more way to curb your sweet tooth. And: it works for me and my clients.

# RULE 12

## LAY OFF *ALL* BOOZE

There are so many reasons that you shouldn't be drinking alcohol while trying to Jumpstart your weight loss. Let me count the ways:

Alcohol—and I mean all that longevity-boosting Chianti as well as spirits and beer—is a central nervous system depressant. You don't ever want that, and you really don't want it now, on your way to the big day!

Booze will make you retain more water and look bloated. Not good for the fit of your dress.

Booze will make your eyes look puffy. Not good for the photos.

And last, booze will alter your metabolism and slow down fat-burning. All-around not good, don't you agree?

Of course, then there's the simple fact that this is a low-calorie three-week diet, and alcohol contains calories that are not accounted for in this program! Here's a look at calorie counts for some popular drinks:

Beer (12 ounces): 150 calories

Light (reduced-calorie) beer (12 ounces): 110 calories

Dark beer (12 ounces): 168 calories

Scotch, vodka, bourbon, gin (1.5 ounces): 100 calories

Dry dessert wine (5 ounces): 198 calories

Sweet dessert wine (5 ounces): 344 calories

Red wine (5 ounces): 105 calories

White wine (5 ounces): 100 calories

Sparkling white wine (5 ounces): 106 calories

What about mixed drinks? Oh, *right*! Check out *this* list:

Bloody Mary (4 ounces): 120 calories

Daiquiri (2.7 ounces): 137 calories

Gin and tonic (7 ounces): 189 calories

Manhattan (2.1 ounces): 132 calories

Margarita (6.3 ounces): 327 calories

Martini (2 ounces): 119 calories

Rum and Coke (12 ounces): 361 calories

Screwdriver (7 ounces): 208 calories

Whiskey sour (3 ounces): 125 calories

Last but not least, it may surprise you that my objection to alcohol while on Jumpstart is less about calorie intake and bloating and eye puffiness (and insulin pathway signaling!) than it is about something much more fundamental . . .

Every now and then, while driving home late at night from a long day at the ranch, I see a line of guys outside the local open-late burger place. All of them fat and, from the looks of it, drunk.

The two states (fat and drunk) are deeply connected—and not because of some complicated metabolic science.

It's because drinking leads to disinhibition, a suspension from your normal rational way of controlling your behavior. That's a fancy way of saying that when you drink alcohol, you let your guard down. You become "disinhibited" to do the right thing. You know, like oversharing about your grooming habits, or giving your number to the random guy you met at the bar, or saying something offensive (or bad for your career, anyway) to your boss at the office party.

Or just outright saying: "Screw that &^%$ Harper, I'm eating that donut!"

Yup, when you drink alcohol it's a slippery slope to raiding the fridge or the drive-through. Or the open-all-night local burger place.

Your Jumpstart program is just three weeks. I know you can say no to booze for that long. You'll feel *so* much better physically and you'll stay in control of those late-night cravings. This is essential: just don't do it!

# RULE 13

------------

## AN ESPRESSO A DAY . . . OR TWO OR THREE

Over the past few years, there has been a spate of research about the health benefits of coffee consumption. It's been linked to everything from better glucose control to lower risk of heart disease and even to healthier cognition and weight loss.

In one study, a group of Japanese civil servants saw an increase in their fat-burning metabolism in conjunction with caffeine consumption. And another study published in that great beach-read known as *Molecular Nutrition and Food Research* concluded: "Dark roast coffee is more effective than light roast coffee in reducing body weight, and in restoring red blood cell vitamin E and glutathione concentrations in healthy volunteers."

"Reducing body weight" is a key positive here. But don't discount the vitamin E and glutathione concentrations. Vitamin E and glutathione boost exercise recovery. A good thing.

In fact, caffeine's main toning-up benefits may come

indirectly—not from simply "revving up" your metabolism. So says a report from the exercise physiology laboratory at the University of Castilla-La Mancha in Spain. The study looked at a common complaint—and physiological reality—of most athletes: in the morning, it's harder to get muscles up to their peak performance than later in the day.

Since many people—if not most—exercise in the morning, and because exercise (both morning and otherwise) is such a key element in the Jumpstart program, let's pay attention. Twelve cyclists were given three different regimens: one with morning caffeine (10 A.M.) followed by exercises (bench presses, squats, and the like), one with a morning placebo followed by the same exercises, and one with an afternoon placebo followed by the same exercise.

Results: "Caffeine ingestion reverses the morning neuromuscular declines in highly resistance-trained men, raising performance to the levels of the afternoon trial."

Translation: Caffeine will make you perform and get the maximal benefits from your Jumpstart regimen!

My preferred delivery system (to use the scientific term) for caffeine and its various constituents is espresso. I prefer it because it makes me less jittery than regular coffee. Per serving, espresso actually has a lot less caffeine than a cup of coffee. And then there's the fundamental reason: drinking espresso makes me think of being in Paris, one of my favorite skinny cities. Let's face it, ordering and sipping espresso feels and looks cool! Feel free to have one before your morning walk. Or pour it in 6 ounces of hot water for an *Americano* if you don't like the intensity of pure espresso. Have several over the course of the day! (You'll see in my day-by-day regimen that I've suggested two points in the day for espresso. You can also have black coffee—or tea.)

## ESPRESSO, S'IL VOUS PLAÎT!

Espresso is meant to be taken black—no milk. Those little serving cups leave no room for adding milk anyway.

Many people drink it without sugar, too. If that describes you, great—black, no sugar it is. But if you (like me) want to cut the bitterness just a tad, go ahead and add half of one raw sugar packet or cube (absolutely no artificial sweetener/sugar substitutes, people!). No more! You don't need anything that might trigger your sweet tooth.

# PART II

# THE JUMPSTART DAY-BY-DAY REGIMEN

Would you "guesstimate" how much medication you should take to reduce your blood pressure? Would you decide for yourself how many reps of leg extensions you should do for physical therapy after a knee operation?

No. I don't think you would. You'd follow the advice of the expert whose advice you sought in the first place. You'd follow that person's *prescription*.

The same should be the case when it comes to meeting your weight goal in advance of your big day—wedding, reunion, party, vacation. You need to follow *my expert prescription* to get you to the altar, high school gym, red carpet, or beach looking your best.

Remember, I've got years of experience with clients, contestants, and *myself,* and there's one other thing I know for sure: the best results come from meticulous planning. Anytime I've had to get ready for a magazine cover shoot (i.e., lose a little weight and tone up quickly!), I've been successful and liked how I looked because I paid particular attention to the details of my diet and exercise for several weeks ahead of time.

But aren't you the lucky one? I've done the work of the next three weeks—the meticulous planning—for you.

The daily plans that follow will hold your hand the whole way. Your daily diet will consist of very simple units of either 275 calories per meal (women) or 400 calories per meal (men). Adhering to Rule 1, each meal will consist of 40 percent protein, 40 percent carbohydrates (mainly from veggies), and 20 percent fat. If you follow my directions, you'll also be getting enough water and electrolyte replacement. Wherever I call for you to drink water or soda water (in 16-ounce increments), know that you can add lemon or lime for flavor. Whenever I call for you to have an espresso or tea, remember—no more than just a half packet or cube of raw sugar; you can add lemon to your tea if you'd like.

I've left only a few decisions up to you:

- You can choose which five days each week you will do your Skinny Moves routine. But you must choose five days!
- You can choose *which* routine you do each day. But you must choose one of them five times a week and a different one each day! You won't need more than some hand weights and a jump rope for five of the routines (so no excuses!), but if you want more variation, try the two routines that require a medicine ball and exercise bands. See Part III for details on what movements and how many reps for each routine.
- The day-by-day regimens that follow prescribe specific recipes for each day, but what's most important is that you eat from my recipes (see Part IV), not which breakfast you eat on what day. If, for instance, you fall in love with my Oatsotto, feel free to have that every day instead of what's shown for the next morning. So long as you choose meals from my recipes for power breakfasts, lean lunches, and thinner dinners, and so long as during week 3 you stay away from recipes that contain fruit, you're all set.

- I've given you specific amounts of water (and other beverages) to drink at each point in the day. You can certainly drink more water than I've prescribed if you want! You can also have more than the one or two espressos listed in the day-to-day instructions.

But that's it—that's all the wiggle room you get and all the wiggle room you need. From morning until night, you will eat, drink, and walk when I say in the pages that follow.

**ATTENTION TO DETAIL!**

As I've said, I've paid attention to the details so you don't have to. But that means you need to pay attention to my prescription! I want you to follow *exactly* the prescribed amounts in each recipe. Half a cup of yogurt is not three-fourths of a cup of yogurt! It's half. You wouldn't take "an extra" blood pressure med, a "tad more" insulin, or just a "pinch" more antibiotic. Right? You know what I mean.

## WEEK 1

### Day 1

*Upon rising:* 16 ounces water, one espresso

*Before breakfast:* 30–45 minutes low-intensity walk or other cardio, then electrolyte replacement in an 8-ounce glass of water (or 8-ounce no-sugar sports drink)

### Breakfast

Quinoa Rancheros

16 ounces water

*After breakfast:* 1,000 mg fish oil, multivitamin, and electrolyte replacement in a 16-ounce glass of water (or 8-ounce no-sugar sports drink)

### Lunch

Roasted Mixed Veggie and Chicken Salad

Espresso or tea

16 ounces water or soda water

1,000 mg fish oil

### Dinner

Mexican Fiesta Fish

16 ounces soda water

1,000 mg fish oil

Optional: herbal tea before bed

**JUMPSTART MOVES:** If this is one of your met-con days, try the Basic AMRAP.

## Day 2

*Upon rising:* 16 ounces water, one espresso

*Before breakfast:* 30–45 minutes low-intensity walk or other cardio, then electrolyte replacement in an 8-ounce glass of water (or 8-ounce no-sugar sports drink)

### Breakfast

Quinoatmeal

16 ounces water

*After breakfast:* 1,000 mg fish oil, multivitamin, and electrolyte replacement in a 16-ounce glass of water (or 8-ounce no-sugar sports drink)

### Lunch

Chicken and Celery Salad

Espresso or tea

16 ounces water or soda water

1,000 mg fish oil

### Dinner

Roasted Mixed Veggies with Turkey Patty

16 ounces water or soda water

1,000 mg fish oil

Optional: herbal tea before bed

**JUMPSTART MOVES:** If this is one of your met-con days, try the Ball Buster.

## Day 3

*Upon rising:* 16 ounces water, one espresso

*Before breakfast:* 30–45 minutes low-intensity walk or other cardio, then electrolyte replacement in an 8-ounce glass of water (or 8-ounce no-sugar sports drink)

### Breakfast

Pizza Toast

16 ounces water

*After breakfast:* 1,000 mg fish oil, multivitamin, and electrolyte replacement in a 16-ounce glass of water (or 8-ounce no-sugar sports drink)

### Lunch

Watermelon Cucumber Salad with Salmon

Espresso or tea

16 ounces water or soda water

1,000 mg fish oil

### Dinner

Herbed Turkey Meatball and Veggie Soup

16 ounces water or soda water

1,000 mg fish oil

Optional: herbal tea before bed

**JUMPSTART MOVES:** If this is one of your met-con days, try the Classic Met-Con.

## Day 4

*Upon rising:* 16 ounces water, one espresso

*Before breakfast:* 30–45 minutes low-intensity walk or other cardio, then electrolyte replacement in an 8-ounce glass of water (or 8-ounce no-sugar sports drink)

### Breakfast

Aspareggus Scramble

16 ounces water

*After breakfast:* 1,000 mg fish oil, multivitamin, and electrolyte replacement in a 16-ounce glass of water (or 8-ounce no-sugar sports drink)

### Lunch

Apple Chicken Salad

Espresso or tea

16 ounces water or soda water

1,000 mg fish oil

### Dinner

Chicken Alla Fresca

16 ounces water or soda water

1,000 mg fish oil

Optional: herbal tea before bed

**JUMPSTART MOVES:** If this is one of your met-con days, try the Medicine Man.

## Day 5

*Upon rising:* 16 ounces water, one espresso

*Before breakfast:* 30–45 minutes low-intensity walk or other cardio, then electrolyte replacement in an 8-ounce glass of water (or 8-ounce no-sugar sports drink)

### Breakfast

Roasted Vegetable Frittata

16 ounces water

*After breakfast:* 1,000 mg fish oil, multivitamin, and electrolyte replacement in a 16-ounce glass of water (or 8-ounce no-sugar sports drink)

### Lunch

Asparagus and Chicken Salad

Espresso or tea

16 ounces water or soda water

1,000 mg fish oil

### Dinner

Jumbo Stir-Fry

16 ounces water or soda water

1,000 mg fish oil

Optional: herbal tea before bed

**JUMPSTART MOVES:** If this is one of your met-con days, try Fleet Feet.

## Day 6

*Upon rising:* 16 ounces water, one espresso

*Before breakfast:* 30–45 minutes low-intensity walk or other cardio, then electrolyte replacement in an 8-ounce glass of water (or 8-ounce no-sugar sports drink)

### Breakfast

Peanut Butter and "Jelly" Oatmeal with Egg White Scramble

16 ounces water

*After breakfast:* 1,000 mg fish oil, multivitamin, and electrolyte replacement in a 16-ounce glass of water (or 8-ounce no-sugar sports drink)

### Lunch

Hearty Salad

Espresso or tea

16 ounces water or soda water

1,000 mg fish oil

### Dinner

Spaghetti Squash Bolognese

16 ounces water or soda water

1,000 mg fish oil

Optional: herbal tea before bed

**JUMPSTART MOVES:** If this is one of your met-con days, try the Band of Death.

## Day 7

*Upon rising:* 16 ounces water, one espresso

*Before breakfast:* 30–45 minutes low-intensity walk or other cardio, then electrolyte replacement in an 8-ounce glass of water (or 8-ounce no-sugar sports drink)

### Breakfast

"Shake and Eggs"

16 ounces water

*After breakfast:* 1,000 mg fish oil, multivitamin, and electrolyte replacement in a 16-ounce glass of water (or 8-ounce no-sugar sports drink)

### Lunch

Tomato-Fennel Salad

Espresso or tea

16 ounces water or soda water

1,000 mg fish oil

### Dinner

Orange and Parsley Fish "Pockets" with Roasted Asparagus and Fennel

16 ounces water or soda water

1,000 mg fish oil

Optional: herbal tea before bed

**JUMPSTART MOVES:** If this is one of your met-con days, try the Body Lift.

# WEEK 2

## Day 1

*Upon rising:* 16 ounces water, one espresso

*Before breakfast:* 30–45 minutes low-intensity walk or other cardio, then electrolyte replacement in an 8-ounce glass of water (or 8-ounce no-sugar sports drink)

### Breakfast

Scrambled Pasta

16 ounces water

*After breakfast:* 1,000 mg fish oil, multivitamin, and electrolyte replacement in a 16-ounce glass of water (or 8-ounce no-sugar sports drink)

### Lunch

Kale Salad

Espresso or tea

16 ounces water or soda water

1,000 mg fish oil

### Dinner

Halibut "Tacos" with Tropical Salsa

16 ounces water or soda water

1,000 mg fish oil

Optional: herbal tea before bed

**JUMPSTART MOVES:** If this is one of your met-con days, try the Basic AMRAP.

## Day 2

*Upon rising:* 16 ounces water, one espresso

*Before breakfast:* 30–45 minutes low-intensity walk or other cardio, then electrolyte replacement in an 8-ounce glass of water (or 8-ounce no-sugar sports drink)

### Breakfast

Turkey Scramble

16 ounces water

*After breakfast:* 1,000 mg fish oil, multivitamin, and electrolyte replacement in a 16-ounce glass of water (or 8-ounce no-sugar sports drink)

### Lunch

Roasted Tomato Salad

Espresso or tea

16 ounces water or soda water

1,000 mg fish oil

### Dinner

Green Cauliflower Soup

16 ounces water or soda water

1,000 mg fish oil

Optional: herbal tea before bed

**JUMPSTART MOVES:** If this is one of your met-con days, try the Band of Death.

## Day 3

*Upon rising:* 16 ounces water, one espresso

*Before breakfast:* 30–45 minutes low-intensity walk or other cardio, then electrolyte replacement in an 8-ounce glass of water (or 8-ounce no-sugar sports drink)

### Breakfast

Yogurt with Tropical Fruit

16 ounces water

*After breakfast:* 1,000 mg fish oil, multivitamin, and electrolyte replacement in a 16-ounce glass of water (or 8-ounce no-sugar sports drink)

### Lunch

Roasted Vegetable Salad with Turkey

Espresso or tea

16 ounces water or soda water

1,000 mg fish oil

### Dinner

Shrimp Skimpy

16 ounces water or soda water

1,000 mg fish oil

Optional: herbal tea before bed

**JUMPSTART MOVES:** If this is one of your met-con days, try the Classic Met-Con.

## Day 4

*Upon rising:* 16 ounces water, one espresso
*Before breakfast:* 30–45 minutes low-intensity walk or other cardio, then electrolyte replacement in an 8-ounce glass of water (or 8-ounce no-sugar sports drink)

### Breakfast

Spicy Asparagus and Quinoa
16 ounces water
*After breakfast:* 1,000 mg fish oil, multivitamin, and electrolyte replacement in a 16-ounce glass of water (or 8-ounce no-sugar sports drink)

### Lunch

Pesto Chicken Salad
Espresso or tea
16 ounces water or soda water
1,000 mg fish oil

### Dinner

Steak and Pesto "Potatoes" with Roasted Asparagus
16 ounces water or soda water
1,000 mg fish oil
Optional: herbal tea before bed

**JUMPSTART MOVES:** If this is one of your met-con days, try the Ball Buster.

## Day 5

*Upon rising:* 16 ounces water, one espresso

*Before breakfast:* 30–45 minutes low-intensity walk or other cardio, then electrolyte replacement in an 8-ounce glass of water (or 8-ounce no-sugar sports drink)

### Breakfast

Pasta with Pesto Eggs

16 ounces water

*After breakfast:* 1,000 mg fish oil, multivitamin, and electrolyte replacement in a 16-ounce glass of water (or 8-ounce no-sugar sports drink)

### Lunch

Chopped Salad

Espresso or tea

16 ounces water or soda water

1,000 mg fish oil

### Dinner

Mango Chicken

16 ounces water or soda water

1,000 mg fish oil

Optional: herbal tea before bed

**JUMPSTART MOVES:** If this is one of your met-con days, try the Medicine Man.

## Day 6

*Upon rising:* 16 ounces water, one espresso

*Before breakfast:* 30–45 minutes low-intensity walk or other cardio, then electrolyte replacement in an 8-ounce glass of water (or 8-ounce no-sugar sports drink)

### Breakfast

Applesauce Oatmeal with a Side of Green Eggs

16 ounces water

*After breakfast:* 1,000 mg fish oil, multivitamin, and electrolyte replacement in a 16-ounce glass of water (or 8-ounce no-sugar sports drink)

### Lunch

Buffalo Chicken Salad

Espresso or tea

16 ounces water or soda water

1,000 mg fish oil

### Dinner

Eggplant Chili

16 ounces water or soda water

1,000 mg fish oil

Optional: herbal tea before bed

**JUMPSTART MOVES:** If this is one of your met-con days, try the Body Lift.

## Day 7

*Upon rising:* 16 ounces water, one espresso

*Before breakfast:* 30–45 minutes low-intensity walk or other cardio, then electrolyte replacement in an 8-ounce glass of water (or 8-ounce no-sugar sports drink)

### Breakfast

Cucumber-Blueberry Shake with a Side of Eggs

16 ounces water

*After breakfast:* 1,000 mg fish oil, multivitamin, and electrolyte replacement in a 16-ounce glass of water (or 8-ounce no-sugar sports drink)

### Lunch

Taco Salad

Espresso or tea

16 ounces water or soda water

1,000 mg fish oil

### Dinner

Spicy Roasted Chicken with Veggies

16 ounces water or soda water

1,000 mg fish oil

Optional: herbal tea before bed

**JUMPSTART MOVES:** If this is one of your met-con days, try Fleet Feet.

## WEEK 3

### Day 1

*Upon rising:* 16 ounces water, one espresso
*Before breakfast:* 30–45 minutes low-intensity walk or other cardio, then electrolyte replacement in an 8-ounce glass of water (or 8-ounce no-sugar sports drink)

### Breakfast

Ratatouille Scramble
16 ounces water
*After breakfast:* 1,000 mg fish oil, multivitamin, and electrolyte replacement in a 16-ounce glass of water (or 8-ounce no-sugar sports drink)

### Lunch

Not-So-FAToosh
Espresso or tea
16 ounces water or soda water
1,000 mg fish oil

### Dinner

Chicken Ratatouille
16 ounces water or soda water
1,000 mg fish oil
Optional: herbal tea before bed

**JUMPSTART MOVES:** If this is one of your met-con days, try Fleet Feet.

## Day 2

*Upon rising:* 16 ounces water, one espresso

*Before breakfast:* 30–45 minutes low-intensity walk or other cardio, then electrolyte replacement in an 8-ounce glass of water (or 8-ounce no-sugar sports drink)

### Breakfast

Spanish Scramble

16 ounces water

*After breakfast:* 1,000 mg fish oil, multivitamin, and electrolyte replacement in a 16-ounce glass of water (or 8-ounce no-sugar sports drink)

### Lunch

Gazpacho Shrimp Salad

Espresso or tea

16 ounces water or soda water

1,000 mg fish oil

### Dinner

Gourmet Pork "Chop"

16 ounces water or soda water

1,000 mg fish oil

Optional: herbal tea before bed

**JUMPSTART MOVES:** If this is one of your met-con days, try the Classic Met-Con.

## Day 3

*Upon rising:* 16 ounces water, one espresso

*Before breakfast:* 30–45 minutes low-intensity walk or other cardio, then electrolyte replacement in an 8-ounce glass of water (or 8-ounce no-sugar sports drink)

### Breakfast

Sweet Potato Hash

16 ounces water

*After breakfast:* 1,000 mg fish oil, multivitamin, and electrolyte replacement in a 16-ounce glass of water (or 8-ounce no-sugar sports drink)

### Lunch

Chicken Cucumber Salad

Espresso or tea

16 ounces water or soda water

1,000 mg fish oil

### Dinner

Mediterranean Salad

16 ounces water or soda water

1,000 mg fish oil

Optional: herbal tea before bed

**JUMPSTART MOVES:** If this is one of your met-con days, try the Ball Buster.

## Day 4

*Upon rising:* 16 ounces water, one espresso

*Before breakfast:* 30–45 minutes low-intensity walk or other cardio, then electrolyte replacement in an 8-ounce glass of water (or 8-ounce no-sugar sports drink)

### Breakfast

Stuffed Tomato

16 ounces water

*After breakfast:* 1,000 mg fish oil, multivitamin, and electrolyte replacement in a 16-ounce glass of water (or 8-ounce no-sugar sports drink)

### Lunch

Ratatouille Salad

Espresso or tea

16 ounces water or soda water

1,000 mg fish oil

### Dinner

Chicken and Zucchini Pouch

16 ounces water or soda water

1,000 mg fish oil

Optional: herbal tea before bed

**JUMPSTART MOVES:** If this is one of your met-con days, try the Band of Death.

## Day 5

---

*Upon rising:* 16 ounces water, one espresso

*Before breakfast:* 30–45 minutes low-intensity walk or other cardio, then electrolyte replacement in an 8-ounce glass of water (or 8-ounce no-sugar sports drink)

### Breakfast

Quinoaquiles

16 ounces water

*After breakfast:* 1,000 mg fish oil, multivitamin, and electrolyte replacement in a 16-ounce glass of water (or 8-ounce no-sugar sports drink)

### Lunch

Red Cabbage Slaw and Steak

Espresso or tea

16 ounces water or soda water

1,000 mg fish oil

### Dinner

Herbed Chicken with Red Pepper

16 ounces water or soda water

1,000 mg fish oil

Optional: herbal tea before bed

**JUMPSTART MOVES:** If this is one of your met-con days, try Fleet Feet.

## Day 6

*Upon rising:* 16 ounces water, one espresso

*Before breakfast:* 30–45 minutes low-intensity walk or other cardio, then electrolyte replacement in an 8-ounce glass of water (or 8-ounce no-sugar sports drink)

### Breakfast

Shrimp and "Grits"

16 ounces water

*After breakfast:* 1,000 mg fish oil, multivitamin, and electrolyte replacement in a 16-ounce glass of water (or 8-ounce no-sugar sports drink)

### Lunch

Jolly Green Salmon

Espresso or tea

16 ounces water or soda water

1,000 mg fish oil

### Dinner

Swiss Chard and Cabbage Stir-Fry

16 ounces water or soda water

1,000 mg fish oil

Optional: herbal tea before bed

**JUMPSTART MOVES:** If this is one of your met-con days, try the Basic AMRAP.

## Day 7

---

*Upon rising:* 16 ounces water, one espresso

*Before breakfast:* 30–45 minutes low-intensity walk or other cardio, then electrolyte replacement in an 8-ounce glass of water (or 8-ounce no-sugar sports drink)

### Breakfast

Oatsotto

16 ounces water

*After breakfast:* 1,000 mg fish oil, multivitamin, and electrolyte replacement in a 16-ounce glass of water (or 8-ounce no-sugar sports drink)

### Lunch

Confetti Salad

Espresso or tea

16 ounces water or soda water

1,000 mg fish oil

### Dinner

Gourmet Turkey Burger

16 ounces water or soda water

1,000 mg fish oil

Optional: herbal tea before bed

**JUMPSTART MOVES:** If this is one of your met-con days, try the Body Lift.

# PART III

# THE JUMPSTART MOVES

On fifteen of the next twenty-one days (again, days of your choice each week), you'll be doing some intense exercise for fifteen to twenty minutes. You remember that part of the program, right? See Rule 7 if your memory has failed you!

As I mentioned earlier, my Jumpstart Moves put you through metabolic conditioning, or met-con for short. I've created seven perfect routines—what I like to call "packages"—for you to choose from. These are discrete regimens designed to give you an overall tone and polish by the end of the three-week program, but as I've mentioned before, you can mix up the order of the packages if you like. Just be sure to do five different packages over the course of the week.

All you need for five of these exercise packages are some hand weights (or a kettlebell) and a jump rope. I've offered some more advanced versions that use a medicine ball and exercise bands (though you can substitute a dumbbell or hand weight for the medicine ball). If you don't have that extra equipment, notice that there are still plenty of packages that don't require them. No excuses here!

As you complete each package, write down your performance—

the time it took you to complete it, how many rounds or reps you did, and so on. I want you to see your own progress. By week 3, you'll be impressed with yourself!

## IMAGINING YOUR STRENGTH AND POWER

When doing my met-con exercises, I want you to keep the following in mind: use your *middle-line for strength,* and your *hips for power.*

What do I mean by that? Simple. When you do, say, a sit-up, I want you to focus on an imaginary line you might draw from your chin down to your pelvis. Keep it pulled inward as you go through the exercise, literally using the contraction to lift you up. Or, take the standard push-up. Again, as you push yourself up, contract your abs. For each movement, contract the midline as you perform the part of the exercise that requires the most strength, then relax the abs. You'll get it.

Hips for power? That's right. This you'll experience whenever you do a squat properly. With legs apart and back straight, sink down *into your heels,* arms out, butt back, and then push down into your heels as you come up. Feel that? You're using those big muscles in your legs and glutes to power your whole body upward.

Let me now take you, package by package, exercise by exercise, through the Jumpstart Moves.

Ready? You'd better be. Swimsuit season is coming, sister!

## PACKAGE 1: THE BASIC AMRAP

20 sit-ups

15 air squats

10 push-ups

Repeat this sequence for 20 minutes.

Mark down how many complete rounds plus any additional
rounds you do.

AMRAP stands for "as many rounds as possible." Do 20 sit-ups, 15 air squats, and 10 push-ups, and repeat the entire sequence as many times as you can in 20 minutes. When 20 minutes are up, write down how many rounds you were able to finish.

This is one of my most basic (hence its name) and effective met-con sequences. Like all of the Jumpstart Moves, it emphasizes the use of your own body weight. You are doing only three moves— sit-ups, air squats, and push-ups. I want you to get 'em right, which is why I've given such a detailed description. Read this through before beginning. (In fact, read *all* of the explanations in each package before commencing.)

## Sit-Ups

When it comes to abs, slower is better. And concentrate on your form! Make sure to keep your lower back pressed into the floor. Always! You never want to pull your head up, so you'll see that I'm not going to let your hands get near your neck! The lift should come from your abs. That's your sit-up! It's the passport to a better bridal body, slimmer swimsuit shape, and a hot reunion figure.

1. Lie on your back with your arms extended above your head and close to your ears. Press the soles of your feet together and let your knees fall open. Make sure to press your lower back into the floor. I want you to make that connection to the floor and hold it.
2. Lift your torso up off the floor and touch your fingers to the ground in front of your toes, exhale, hold the position, and then lower your head back down. That's one!

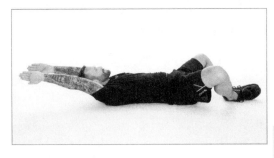

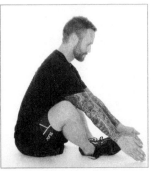

## Air Squats

The air squat for strength and balance is one of the fundamentals of functional fitness. It's a great fat burner, too.

1. Stand with your feet slightly more than shoulder-width apart with both arms by your sides.
2. Now bend your knees and squat as though sitting down on an imaginary chair and extend your arms out in front of you. Keep your back straight and your knees behind your toes. *Sink into your heels. You're aiming to drop your hips below parallel.*
3. Return to standing position. Remember: think butt—not knees! You're squatting, not kneeling.

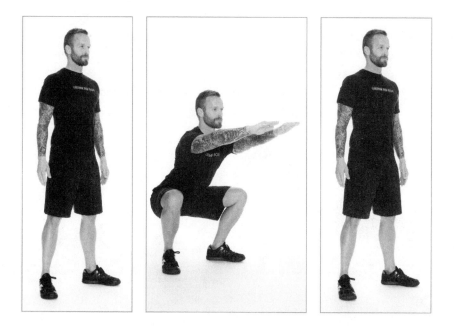

## Push-Ups

The classic push-up, long one of our most familiar exercises, has recently enjoyed a kind of renaissance, and for good reason. People who study exercise single it out as one of the best indicators of a person's overall health and fitness. Men should be able to do twenty; women, ten. Make those minimums your goals for each repetition.

I want you to think about two things as you go through this. One, range of motion. By that I mean I want you to try to bring your chest *as close to the ground as you can* with each rep. Two, I want you to center your attention on your core—that midline we talked about before. Contract your abs and glutes. If you want them tight—you gotta tighten 'em!

1. Get in "push-up position"—that, at least, should be familiar. Keep your back flat, and position your hands just below your shoulders.

2. Slowly lower your chest to the floor, keeping your neck as relaxed as possible. Hold yourself there for a second, then push back up—as if you are pushing your hands through the floor! Keep your abs tight, and do it again.

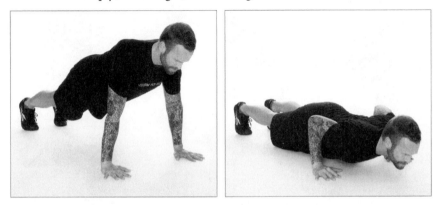

## PACKAGE 2: THE BALL BUSTER

10 weight swings
10 goblet squats
10 sumo deadlifts

This package is the first of a series of weighted movement regimens, in this case using a hand weight or kettlebell. If using the former, pick a weight that's heavy enough to get your attention, but not so heavy that you can't finish at least the first round of each exercise.

In this package, I want you to do As Many Rounds As Possible (AMRAP) in 15 minutes. Keep track of how many rounds you finish.

## Weight Swing

This exercise is good for overall conditioning, but you should feel the effort and stretch most in your core. Remember to use a weight that feels challenging.

1. Stand with your feet a little more than shoulder-width apart and the weight in your hands in front of you. Keep your back straight, shoulders relaxed.
2. Bending your knees slightly for stabilization but keeping your arms straight, lift the weight in one movement above your head.
3. Bring the weight gently back down in front of you and stand up straight again in the start position. You are now ready to do it again.

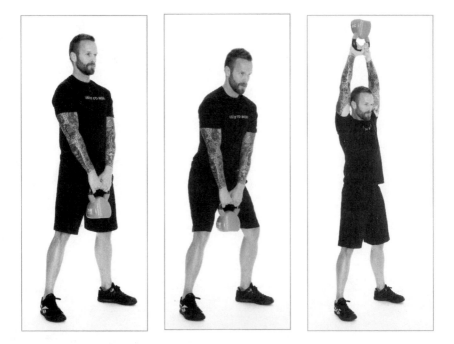

## Goblet Squats

This exercise is a variation on the air squat in the Basic package. The difference here, of course, is the added weight.

1. Stand with your feet slightly more than shoulder-width apart, holding the weight or kettlebell with both hands in front of your chest. Think altar boy with chalice. Your elbows should be pointing downward.
2. Now bend your knees and squat as though sitting down on an imaginary chair while holding the weight steady at your chest. Keep your back straight and your knees behind your toes. *Sink into your heels. You're aiming to drop your hips below parallel.*
3. Rise back up, and do it again.

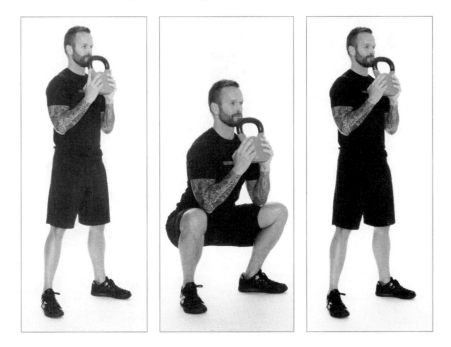

## Sumo Deadlifts

1. Start with your feet apart and the weight in front of you on the floor. Keeping your back straight (no hunching over), squat down, pick up the weight with both hands, and, rising to a full standing position, pull the weight up to your chin. Grimace if you like.
2. Now lower the kettlebell or dumbbell back to the starting position as you squat back down and repeat.

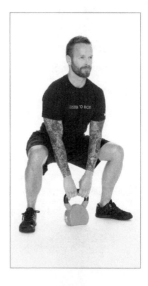

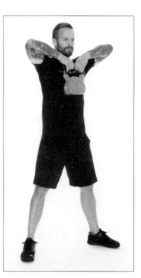

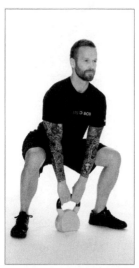

## PACKAGE 3: THE CLASSIC MET-CON

Do five rounds of these exercises for time:

10 burpees
15 chair dips
25 jump ropes, with real or imaginary rope

Note down how long it took you to finish these exercises.

## Burpee

I've talked about the burpee before (see Rule 7), but let's make sure you get it right—because it will change your body if you do!

1. Start out standing with your arms by your sides.
2. Now drop into the squat position and place your hands on the ground in front of you. Count 1.
3. In one quick move, jump your feet back to assume that classic plank position (as at the start of a push-up or a plank in yoga). Count 2.
4. Drop your chest and hips down to the floor. Count 3.
5. Now, in one motion, return to the squat position. Count 4 . . .
6. . . . and then jump straight up into the air, throwing your arms up above your head. Count 5.

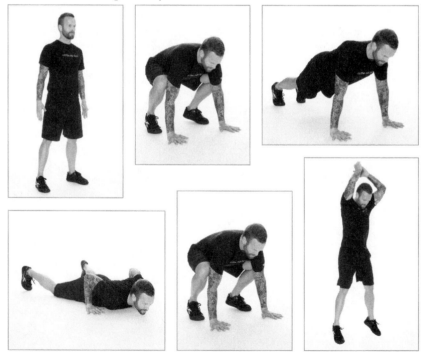

## Chair Dips

Chair dips are a perfect complement to burpees. You'll need a stable chair or bench for this one.

1. With your hands placed on a chair or bench behind you (arms firm and straight), extend your legs in front of you, keeping your feet together.
2. Now "dip" your body by bending at your elbows until they form a 90-degree angle.
3. Then push yourself back up to your original position, so that your arms are straight and supporting your weight again.

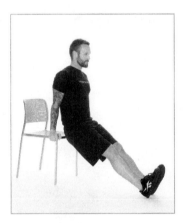 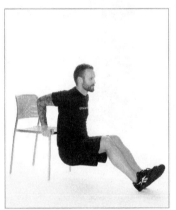

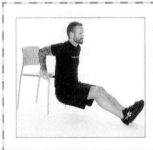

To make this exercise a little more challenging, move your feet out a little farther from your body so that when you "dip," your legs will do less work . . . and your arms will do more!

## Jump Rope

Everyone knows how to jump rope—right? I hope so! Keep in mind that you do not need a fancy or expensive jump rope. In fact, you can use an imaginary one (though having an actual rope to jump over and turn will make you work a little harder)!

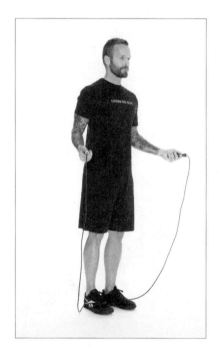

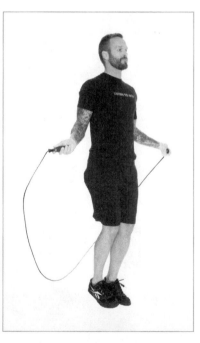

## PACKAGE 4: THE MEDICINE MAN

This package requires a medicine ball but you can substitute a dumbbell or hand weight. Do one round of these, all with a medicine ball or weight, and note down your time:

> 20 medicine ball push-ups
> 20 medicine ball sit-ups
> 20 medicine ball squats
> 20 no-wall balls
> 20 medicine ball burpees

---

**HOW MUCH WEIGHT?**

How do you know if you're using the right weight? Pick it up and play with it a little—see how it feels. If it is unreasonably heavy, get a lighter one. Check out a few moves before your workout. Do you *really* grimace when doing a squat? Can your wrists handle the pressure for the burpee? Maybe you need a slightly lighter weight. Leave the weight out if it prevents you from doing the regimen. But remember—adding a weight or medicine ball maximizes the effectiveness of these moves!

## Medicine Ball Push-Ups

When doing this move, keep the push-up basics in mind: back flat and abs pulled in. Common sense here, too: if using the ball or weight is simply too difficult, do regular push-ups. But add an extra push-up or two to make up for the lack of ball or weight!

1.  You need to get into the traditional plank position that is the start of a push-up, the difference here being that you will be balancing your hands on the ball (or weights) in front of you.
2.  Now lower yourself down until your chest touches the ball (or weights).
3.  Push back up.

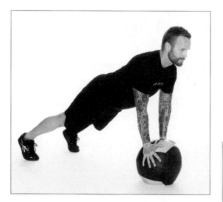

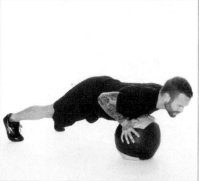

## Medicine Ball Sit-Ups

1. Lie down on the floor, with the ball or weight positioned at arm's length behind your head. Put your feet together, bend your knees, and then let them fall apart. Extend your arms back and pick up the ball (or weight).

2. Keeping your abs tucked and your lower back resting on the ground, swing the ball forward as you rise all the way up, reaching between your legs and, if possible, touching the floor at your feet.

3. Now roll back down. Do these slowly, and do them correctly. It's worth it.

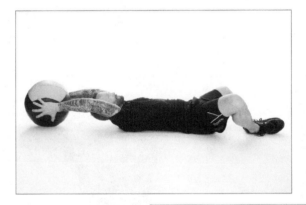

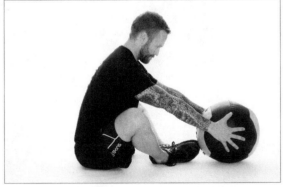

## Medicine Ball Squats

You'll do these *almost* the same way you do a regular squat, so see page 81 for the correct form.

1.  Standing with your legs shoulder-width apart, hold the medicine ball or weight behind your head, with elbows pointed up toward the ceiling or sky.
2.  Squat to a sitting position, sinking into your heels. Aim to drop your hips below parallel.
3.  Rise back up and repeat.

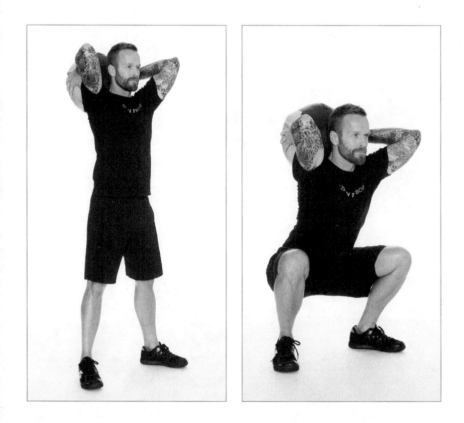

## No-Wall Balls

Don't try this exercise with weights—it really should be done only with a medicine ball.

1. Stand with your feet shoulder-width apart and hold the ball to your chin, with elbows pointing down at the ground.
2. Squat down as low as you can to the floor, keeping your back straight and the ball in place in front of you. Aim to drop your hips below parallel.
3. Now stand up and extend your arms straight up above you and toss the ball gently into the air. Catch the ball, and return to the start position. That's one!

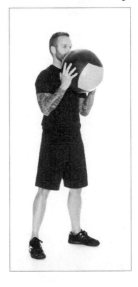
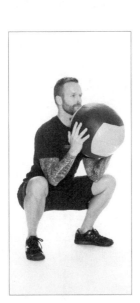
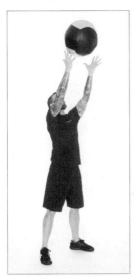

## Medicine Ball Burpee

Like the medicine ball push-up, this is a demanding exercise. If you don't have a ball or weights or if the exercise is too hard for you, do a regular burpee. This is a move worth working toward, perhaps during week 3, when you're feeling the benefits of other Jumpstart packages.

1. Stand with your legs apart. Hold the ball or weight in front of you at the waist.
2. Bend your knees and bend at the hips to place the ball on the ground in front of you. Keep your back flat—no hunching over!
3. While still holding the ball between your hands, jump your legs back into a plank position, keeping your arms straight and elbows locked.
4. Now bend your arms to do a push-up on the ball or weight. Keep your back straight!
5. Jump your legs forward and rise back up, lifting the ball back off the ground and into the starting position.

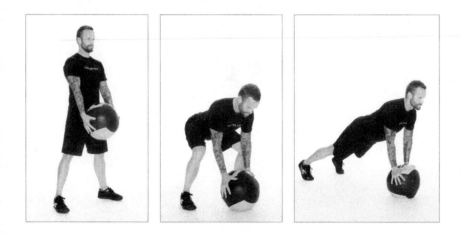

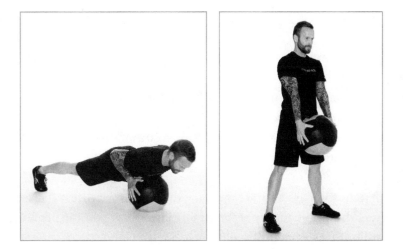

As with the medicine ball push-up, do a trial run to make sure your wrists can withstand the pressure: do one push-up with your knees on the ground. I don't want you to hurt yourself.

## PACKAGE 5: FLEET FEET

Do five rounds:

> 5 minutes—run or walk as fast as you can
> 1 minute—recovery walk
> 5 rounds of AMRAP or AMRAP in 20 minutes
> Note: morning walk also required

All right you guys, why are we doing this? My experience is that as my clients get fitter, they become more inspired by more aggressive cardio. That's what this is—in small, bite-size amounts. The Fleet Feet routine will rev up your metabolism and really wake you up.

## PACKAGE 6: THE BAND OF DEATH

> 20 band pulls
> 20 band presses
> 20 band thrusts
> Do 5 rounds as fast as you can, make a note of your time.

The elastic exercise band is another effective, portable, and inexpensive tool you can use in dozens of ways. You can use it any time of day, and you don't even have to change your clothes to do it. Do these exercises in your office, hotel room, or, of course, your TV room. Remember to time yourself.

## Band Pull

This is a great way to work your upper back, which will be on display in a wedding gown or swimsuit, so get it right and do it often.

1.  Secure the band in front of you by looping it through a couple of heavy kettlebells if you have them, or around a pole, the doorknob of a closed door, or sofa leg (something heavy and secure enough to stay put while you exercise).
2.  Holding each handle of the band, stand with your feet shoulder-width apart and your knees slightly bent. Pull the bands toward your chest, keeping your elbows tucked and pointing behind you. When you have the bands pulled as far back as you can, imagine you are squeezing an imaginary finger at the center of your back.
3.  Slowly go back to the arms-extended position. Repeat.

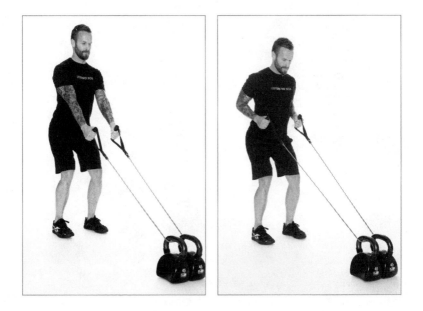

## Band Press

Do ten band presses with one leg bent, then do ten more with the other leg bent.

1. The setup for this is the opposite of the Band Pull. The bands should be looped around or through something secure behind you this time.
2. Kneel down on one knee, keeping the other bent at a 90 degree angle in front of you. Hold the ends of the bands at chest level with your elbows pointing behind you.
3. Now press your arms straight out, straightening your elbows and holding the bands steady in front of you. This sort of looks like a vertical push-up!

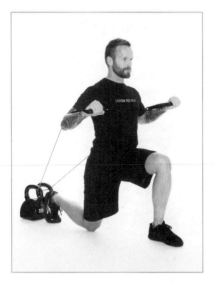
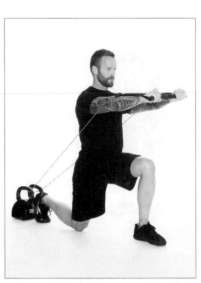

## Band Thrusts

I love band thrusts! They are basically super-effective squats.

1. Stand on the middle of the band with your feet hip-width apart. Squat down (keeping your back straight and butt back!) and hold one end of the band in each hand as though you are going to show off your biceps.
2. Now stand up and straighten your arms overhead.
3. Lower them to your original position as you return to a squat.

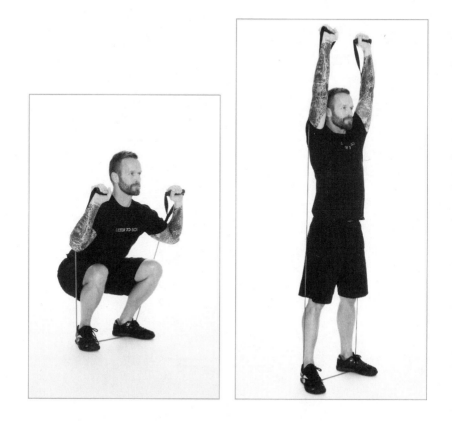

## PACKAGE 7: THE BODY LIFT

20 high-knee tucks

10 mountain climbers in push-up position

20 lateral jumps

20 sit-ups

Do as many rounds as possible in 12 minutes.

## High-Knee Tucks

In theory, this movement is very simple. Still, let's make sure your form is correct.

1. Stand with your legs comfortably apart, and let your arms hang by your sides.
2. Pushing off your toes, jump up vertically and grab your shins with your hands at the height of your leap.
3. Release your knees, come back down to the ground, and get ready to leap again.

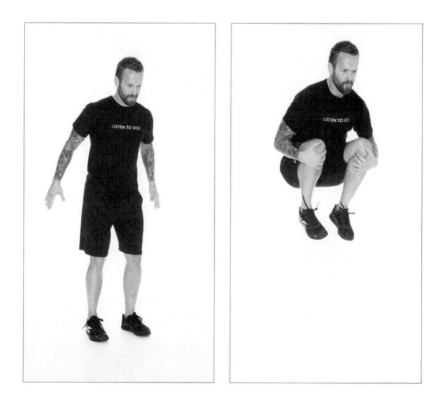

## Mountain Climber in Push-Up Position

See page 82 for the correct starting form for a push-up. Do this exercise at the fastest clip you can without sacrificing form.

1. From the starting plank/push-up position, bring one knee toward your head, and place your foot on the floor to the outside of your hand.
2. Extend your leg back to the starting position.
3. Now do the other side.

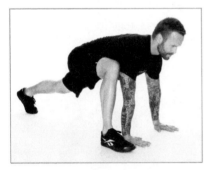 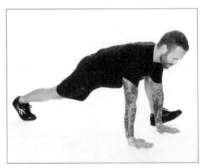

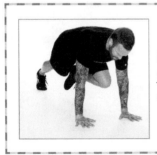

For an easier modification to this exercise, just bring one knee at a time up to your chest.

## Lateral Jumps

You need to create a sense of a line over which you'll jump from side to side for this one. You can use almost anything for this. If you have a jump rope, you can create a line by doubling the rope up and laying it on the floor next to you.

1. Stand with your feet together on one side of the line you've created on the floor.
2. Jump over the line laterally, landing softly on your feet and bending your knees to absorb your descending weight. Jump back. That's one.

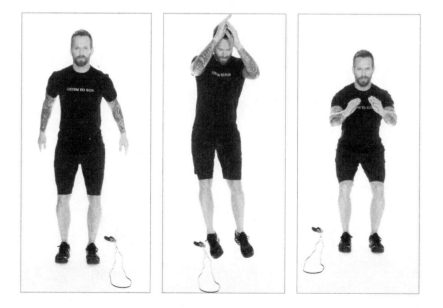

## Sit-Ups

Let me remind you of the proper form. Get going! That bathing suit awaits.

1. Lie on your back with your arms extended above your head and close to your ears. Press the soles of your feet together and let your knees fall open. Make sure to press your lower back into the floor. I want you to make that connection to the floor and hold it.
2. Lift your torso up off the floor and touch your fingers to the ground in front of your toes, exhale, hold the position, and then lower your head back down. That's one!

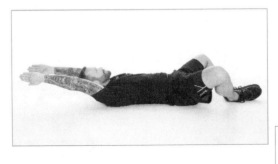

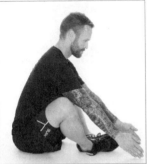

# PART IV

# THE JUMPSTART RECIPES

You've read my Jumpstart Rules, you've considered my menus and exercise routines; now you're about to start cooking some power breakfasts, lean lunches, and thinner dinners. And eating them!

What follows is one recipe in each category for the next twenty-one days. That's twenty-one power breakfasts, twenty-one lean lunches, and twenty-one thinner dinners. In case the math escapes you, that's a total of sixty-three new recipes, laid out in the order you'll get to them in my menus.

All of these recipes adhere to Rule 1 (40/40/20—the magic macronutrient proportions), though because many of your carbs will come from fruits and veggies, the net carbs for many of the lunch and dinner recipes are sometimes fewer than 40 percent carbs. That's okay! Remember, I am letting you eat all the veggies you want during the day, so as long as you follow the no-complex-carbs-after-breakfast rule, you'll be eating exactly as I want you to. And over the course of each day, the total calories will meet the needs of Rule 2 (800 calories for women, 1,200 for men). They will also ensure you don't get too much salt. Yes, that's right—I've thought of everything for you. And you're welcome!

You'll also notice that at the beginning of each week's worth of recipes, I've listed the ingredients (like roasted vegetables and chicken) or sauces (pesto, marinara, pico de gallo, etc.) you should prepare ahead of time and then store for later in the week. Make or chop these basic building blocks in the amounts specified and you'll have what you need for that week. Not only will this advance prep make things easier for you, it's also a great way to improve your chances of staying on this plan. When you come home exhausted from work in the middle of the week, you will have less to do . . . and therefore no excuses for not eating as I say!

---

**HOW TO CALCULATE A MAN'S PORTION**

The recipes that follow all yield the appropriate portions to add up to a woman's 800-calorie day. Remember, men get a little more: 1,200 calories. The math isn't hard! An extra 400 calories per day—the male Jumpstart requirement—works out to 1.5 times the female portion. So if you're a man on this diet, plan accordingly, remembering to increase the amounts in the Prepare Ahead and Store foods.

---

I find that most people want to follow the menus and therefore the recipes in exact order, and they're hesitant to substitute other veggies for the ones specified. Fair enough if that describes you. But when it comes to vegetables, keep an open mind! Brussels sprouts and green beans are great substitutes in recipes that call for asparagus. Take a look at the list of sanctioned vegetables on pages 37 and 38 and be creative.

You can also substitute a recipe you come to love for another if that makes you happy. I *do* want you to be happy! Maybe my Spanish Scramble is what most satisfies you in the morning, or you just can't get enough of my Chicken Ratatouille for dinner. Good—eat what you love. But in week 3, stay away from any recipes that contain fruit (Rule 11).

Last—and this may sound overly basic, but I'll offer some Recipe 101 anyway—before you begin cooking, read through the whole recipe and make sure you have what you need, that you preheat the oven if that's called for, and so forth. None of my recipes are complicated, but it never hurts to get organized ahead of time!

---

**GET YOUR WATER FIX**

Here's an idea: drink your prescribed 16 ounces of water *as you're cooking*. Why not? You're standing there at the counter or stove and though you'll be mixing and stirring a little, you can give your hands and mouth something to do other than nibble on extra ingredients. Have more water (with lemon or lime if you like) or an espresso or tea with your meal, and you'll be that much closer to the total number of ounces you need to pour down your throat each day!

# WEEK 1

*Prepare Ahead and Store*

## Cooked Quinoa

INGREDIENTS
- 1 cup water
- ½ cup quinoa

DIRECTIONS
1. Bring the water to a boil in a small saucepan.
2. Add the quinoa to the boiling water, stir, and reduce the heat to low.
3. Cover and let simmer until cooked and fluffy, about 15 minutes. Turn off heat.
4. Let sit for 5 minutes, then fluff with a fork.

*Note: This will be used in two breakfast recipes.*

NUTRITIONAL INFORMATION PER SERVING
156 calories, 6g protein, 27g carbs, 3g fat, 3g fiber

## Roasted Chicken Breast

INGREDIENTS

Olive oil spray

7 4-ounce skinless, boneless chicken breasts

Cracked black pepper

DIRECTIONS

1. Preheat the oven to 350°F.
2. Spray a baking sheet with olive oil.
3. Lay the chicken breasts on the baking sheet in a single layer.
4. Coat lightly with olive oil spray and cracked pepper.
5. Bake for 15 to 20 minutes or until the juices run clear.

*Note: Each chicken breast will be used individually in meals during the week.*

NUTRITIONAL INFORMATION PER SERVING

134 calories, 25g protein, 0g carbs, 3g fat, 0g fiber

## Roasted Asparagus

INGREDIENTS

16 asparagus spears

Olive oil spray

Cracked black pepper (optional)

DIRECTIONS

1. Preheat the oven to 425°F.
2. Spread the asparagus on a baking sheet, coat evenly with a spritz of olive oil, sprinkle with black pepper if desired, and toss. Rearrange the asparagus in a single layer.
3. Roast for 10 minutes.

*Note: This recipe will be used in two meals during the week.*

NUTRITIONAL INFORMATION PER SERVING

26 calories, 3g protein, 5g carbs, 0g fat, 3g fiber

## Roasted Mixed Veggies

### INGREDIENTS

2 zucchini

2 yellow squash

1 bell pepper

½ red onion

3 green onions (scallions), roughly chopped and using both green
and white parts

Olive oil spray

Cracked black pepper

¼ cup roughly torn basil leaves

### DIRECTIONS

1. Preheat the oven to 425°F.
2. Cut all vegetables into ⅓-inch dice and place in a single layer
   in a baking dish.
3. Coat evenly with a light spritz of olive oil and sprinkle with
   pepper. Toss to coat veggies with the oil.
4. Roast for 20 minutes.
5. Remove from the oven and mix in the basil; it will wilt from
   the heat of the vegetables.
6. Let cool, then store in an airtight container in the fridge.

*Note: This recipe will be used in three meals during the week.*

### NUTRITIONAL INFORMATION PER SERVING

80 calories, 4g protein, 17g carbs, 1g fat, 4g fiber

## Bob's Marinara

------------------------------------------------

### INGREDIENTS

1 tablespoon extra-virgin olive oil
1 small yellow onion, chopped
2 garlic cloves, crushed
1 cup low-sodium vegetable broth
32 ounces low-sodium canned crushed tomatoes
1 bay leaf
¼ cup roughly chopped fresh basil

### DIRECTIONS

1. In a large pot, heat the oil over medium-high heat. Add the onion and sauté until translucent, about 10 minutes. Add the garlic and stir.
2. Add the broth, tomatoes, and bay leaf. Simmer, uncovered, over low heat until the sauce thickens, about 1 hour.
3. Remove and discard the bay leaf. Stir in the basil.

*Note: Serving size is ½ cup; serves 8. This recipe will be used in two meals during the week. Feel free to freeze the rest or share with friends and neighbors.*

### NUTRITIONAL INFORMATION PER SERVING

62 calories, 2g protein, 11 carbs, 2g fat, 3g fiber

## Pico de Gallo

INGREDIENTS

4 plum tomatoes, chopped

¼ cup finely chopped red onion

1 to 2 tablespoons finely chopped fresh cilantro

1 small jalapeño pepper, seeded and chopped

1 small garlic clove, crushed

½ tablespoon fresh lime juice

DIRECTIONS

Lightly toss all ingredients and store in an airtight container in the fridge.

*Note: This recipe will be used in two meals during the week.*

NUTRITIONAL INFORMATION PER SERVING

39 calories, 2g protein, 9g carbs, 0g fat, 2g fiber

## Spaghetti Squash

### INGREDIENTS

½ spaghetti squash, cut lengthwise

### DIRECTIONS

1. Scoop out the seeds. Place in a deep bowl with an inch of water and microwave for 6 minutes per pound. Let cool.
2. When the squash is cool enough to handle, scrape the flesh (horizontally) into strands using a fork.

*Note: This will be used in two dishes this week. Serving size is 1 cup.*

### NUTRITIONAL INFORMATION PER SERVING

42 calories, 1g protein, 110g carbs, 0g fat, 2g fiber

---

**CHOP AHEAD AND STORE**

**1 large bunch of celery**
Slice diagonally. Reserve the leaves as well.

**½ watermelon (yield 3 cups cubed)**
Cut into 1-inch cubes.

**2 bunches of Swiss chard (yield 5 cups chopped)**
Remove leaves from stem and ribs, and chop into big pieces. Store with a slightly damp paper towel.

**2 large heads of broccoli (yield 6 cups chopped)**
Chop roughly.

**1 head of green cabbage**
Shred.

*Week 1 Power Breakfasts*

## Quinoa Rancheros

### INGREDIENTS

Olive oil spray

3 cups chopped fresh spinach

5 egg whites, lightly beaten

½ cup pico de gallo

⅓ cup cooked quinoa

¼ avocado, sliced

### DIRECTIONS

1. Heat a medium skillet over medium-high heat. Spray the hot pan with olive oil. Add the spinach and cook until wilted. Set aside on a paper towel to absorb the liquid.
2. Respray the pan and scramble the egg whites. Toss in the salsa and spinach to heat through.
3. Place on top of the quinoa. Add avocado and enjoy.

### NUTRITIONAL INFORMATION PER SERVING

270 calories, 26g protein, 24g carbs, 7g fat, 6g fiber

## Quinoatmeal with Eggs

### INGREDIENTS

⅓ cup cooked quinoa

½ cup unsweetened almond milk

¾ cup fresh blueberries

1 tablespoon ground flaxseed

Olive oil spray

5 egg whites, lightly beaten

Cracked black pepper

### DIRECTIONS

1. Mix the quinoa and almond milk in a small pot.
2. Heat through on the stove over medium heat (or in a microwave for about 45 seconds).
3. Top with berries and flaxseed.
4. Heat a small skillet over medium-high heat and spray with olive oil.
5. Add the egg whites and black pepper and scramble. Serve alongside the quinoatmeal.

### NUTRITIONAL INFORMATION PER SERVING

283 calories, 24g protein, 28g carbs, 6g fat, 5g fiber

## Pizza Toast

INGREDIENTS

1 slice of Ezekiel bread
4 ounces no-salt sliced turkey breast
¼ cup Bob's marinara
2 cups chopped fresh spinach, wilted
½ cup finely chopped broccoli
1 tablespoon grated Parmesan cheese

DIRECTIONS

1. Preheat a regular or toaster oven to 350°F.
2. Place the turkey on the bread, then top with the sauce, spinach, broccoli, and Parmesan.
3. Place in the oven and "toast" for 10 minutes.

NUTRITIONAL INFORMATION PER SERVING

272 calories, 27g protein, 27g carbs, 7g fat, 4g fiber

## Aspareggus Scramble

### INGREDIENTS
1 slice of Ezekiel bread
¼ avocado
Olive oil spray
5 egg whites, lightly beaten
8 roasted asparagus spears, chopped
Cracked black pepper
¼ cup berries

### DIRECTIONS
1. Toast the bread and spread with avocado.
2. Heat a medium skillet over medium heat and spray with olive oil. Pour in the whites and scramble, then add the asparagus and a sprinkle of black pepper.
3. Place the scramble on the toast.
4. Eat with a side of berries.

### NUTRITIONAL INFORMATION PER SERVING
277 calories, 26g protein, 25g carbs, 6g fat, 6g fiber

# Roasted Vegetable Frittata

### INGREDIENTS

Olive oil spray

2 cups chopped Swiss chard

⅓ of the roasted mixed veggies

5 egg whites, lightly beaten

Cracked black pepper

¼ avocado, sliced

½ slice of Ezekiel bread, toasted

### DIRECTIONS

1. Preheat the broiler.
2. Coat a small ovenproof skillet with olive oil spray. Cook the chard on the stove over medium-high heat until it wilts. Remove the chard and set aside on a paper towel.
3. In a bowl, mix the roasted vegetables, egg whites, and chard and sprinkle with pepper.
4. Re-coat the pan with a light spritz of olive oil. Pour in the egg and veggie mixture and place over high heat on the stove. Let cook for about 5 minutes, until the sides start to brown.
5. Place under the broiler and let cook through for a few more minutes, until the top begins to bubble and brown.
6. Top with the avocado and serve with toast.

### NUTRITIONAL INFORMATION PER SERVING

276 calories, 26g protein, 25g carbs, 7g fat, 6g fiber

## Peanut Butter and "Jelly" Oatmeal and Egg White Scramble

### INGREDIENTS

¾ to 1 cup water, depending on your preferred oatmeal thickness

½ tablespoon almond butter

Dash of cinnamon

½ cup rolled oats

¼ cup fresh blueberries

5 egg whites, lightly beaten

Olive oil spray

Cracked black pepper

### DIRECTIONS

1. In a small pot, bring the water to a simmer.
2. Add the almond butter and cinnamon and stir until smooth.
3. Add the oatmeal and cook until done, about 5 minutes.
4. Turn off heat and stir in the berries. Set aside while you cook the eggs.
5. Heat a small skillet over medium heat. Spray with olive oil to coat.
6. Pour the egg whites into the skillet, add pepper, and stir to scramble as the whites turn opaque.

### NUTRITIONAL INFORMATION PER SERVING

304 calories, 25g protein, 30g carbs, 7g fat, 5g fiber

## "Shake and Eggs"

INGREDIENTS

2 cups cubed watermelon

¼ cup frozen berries

1 Persian cucumber, sliced

1 cup chopped fresh spinach

¼ cup ground flaxseed

Olive oil spray

5 egg whites, lightly beaten

Cracked black pepper

DIRECTIONS

1. In a blender, blend the watermelon, berries, cucumber, spinach, and flaxseed.
2. Heat a small skillet over medium-high heat and spray with olive oil.
3. Pour the egg whites into the pan, add pepper, and cook until scrambled.
4. Sip the shake with a smile while eating scrambled egg whites.

NUTRITIONAL INFORMATION PER SERVING

268 calories, 24g protein, 26g carbs, 6g fat, 5g fiber

*Week 1 Lean Lunches*

## Roasted Mixed Veggie and Chicken Salad

INGREDIENTS

2 teaspoons fresh lemon juice

2 teaspoons balsamic vinegar

1 teaspoon Dijon mustard

Pinch of cayenne pepper

½ teaspoon olive oil

⅓ of the roasted mixed veggies

½ small apple, thinly sliced

4 cups mixed greens

4 ounces roasted chicken breast, cubed

DIRECTIONS

1. In a small bowl, whisk the lemon juice, balsamic, Dijon, cayenne, and olive oil.
2. Toss the roasted vegetables with the apple, mixed greens, chicken, and vinaigrette.

NUTRITIONAL INFORMATION PER SERVING

278 calories, 26g protein, 16g carbs, 5g fat, 7g fiber

## Chicken and Celery Salad

### INGREDIENTS

1 cup sliced celery, including leaves

½ teaspoon extra-virgin olive oil

2 teaspoons fresh lemon juice

1 tablespoon freshly grated Parmesan cheese

Cracked black pepper

1 medium apple, thinly sliced

4 ounces roasted chicken breast, shredded

2 cups chopped fresh spinach

### DIRECTIONS

Mix all ingredients together.

### NUTRITIONAL INFORMATION PER SERVING

263 calories, 24g protein, 16g carbs, 6g fat, 7g fiber

## Watermelon Cucumber Salad with Salmon

INGREDIENTS

Olive oil spray

4 ounces salmon

1 cup cubed watermelon

2 small Persian cucumbers, diced

4 cups chopped arugula

3 cups chopped mixed greens

1 tablespoon fresh lime juice

Cracked black pepper

DIRECTIONS

1. Heat a small skillet over medium-high heat and spray with olive oil. Cook the salmon for 7 minutes on each side. (You can cook it the night before and store it for the next day's lunch.)

2. Toss the watermelon, cucumbers, arugula, and mixed greens in the lime juice and sprinkle with pepper.

3. Plate the salmon with the salad and enjoy!

NUTRITIONAL INFORMATION PER SERVING

271 calories, 28g protein, 21g carbs, 8g fat, 3g fiber

## Apple Chicken Salad

INGREDIENTS

4 ounces roasted chicken breast, cubed

1 small apple, cut into cubes

1 cup sliced celery

1 small zucchini, cut into cubes

2 tablespoons nonfat Greek yogurt

1 teaspoon finely chopped fresh dill

1 teaspoon fresh lemon juice

3 cups chopped mixed greens

DIRECTIONS

1. In a small bowl, mix the chicken, apple, celery, zucchini, yogurt, dill, and lemon juice.
2. Place on the mixed greens and watch your coworkers drool with envy.

NUTRITIONAL INFORMATION PER SERVING

265 calories, 27g protein, 25g carbs, 4g fat, 7g fiber

## Hearty Salad

INGREDIENTS

- 1 teaspoon extra-virgin olive oil
- 2 teaspoons balsamic vinegar
- 1 teaspoon Dijon mustard
- Cracked black pepper
- 4 ounces roasted chicken breast, cubed
- 1 cup chopped broccoli
- ½ cup shredded cabbage
- ½ cup chopped red bell pepper
- 1 Persian cucumber, chopped
- 3 cups chopped mixed greens

DIRECTIONS

1. Whisk the olive oil, balsamic, Dijon, and cracked pepper in a bowl.
2. Toss with the chicken and veggies.

NUTRITIONAL INFORMATION PER SERVING

262 calories, 27g protein, 16g carbs, 7g fat, 8g fiber

## Asparagus and Chicken Salad

### INGREDIENTS

8 roasted asparagus spears, chopped

2 cups chopped kale

½ cup chopped red bell pepper

2 small radishes, trimmed and very thinly sliced

½ tablespoon grated Parmesan cheese

4 ounces roasted chicken breast, cubed

1 teaspoon fresh lemon juice

½ teaspoon olive oil

### DIRECTIONS

Lightly toss all ingredients for a lunch that will leave you light and airy.

### NUTRITIONAL INFORMATION PER SERVING

244 calories, 28g protein, 18g carbs, 6g fat, 7g fiber

## Tomato-Fennel Salad

### INGREDIENTS

1 teaspoon extra-virgin olive oil

1 tablespoon fresh lemon juice

1 teaspoon red wine vinegar

Cracked black pepper

4 ounces roasted chicken breast, shredded

1 tomato, sliced

¼ fennel bulb, thinly sliced

3 cups chopped mixed greens

### DIRECTIONS

1. Whisk the olive oil, lemon juice, vinegar, and cracked pepper in a bowl.
2. Toss with the chicken and veggies.

### NUTRITIONAL INFORMATION PER SERVING

268 calories, 27g protein, 24g carbs, 8g fat, 7g fiber

*Week 1 Thinner Dinners*

## Mexican Fiesta Fish

### INGREDIENTS
Olive oil spray

2 cups chopped Swiss chard

1 teaspoon extra-virgin olive oil

¼ yellow onion, thinly sliced

1 teaspoon crushed garlic

1½ cups chopped broccoli

4 ounces halibut or cod

1 cup pico de gallo

### DIRECTIONS
1. Coat a skillet with olive oil spray. Set over medium-high heat, add the chard, and cook until wilted. Remove and place in the center of a plate.
2. In the same pan, add olive oil, then the onion, and sauté, stirring occasionally, until translucent. Add the garlic and stir.
3. Add the broccoli and sauté for 2 minutes, stirring occasionally. Push the broccoli to the sides of the pan and place the halibut or cod in the middle.
4. Cook for 5 to 7 minutes on each side, stirring the broccoli around between flips.
5. Style the plate using the chard as the bed for the fish and broccoli. Top the dish with the vitamin-rich salsa.

### NUTRITIONAL INFORMATION PER SERVING
251 calories, 28g protein, 23g carbs, 7g fat, 7g fiber

## Roasted Mixed Veggies with Turkey Patty

### INGREDIENTS

4 ounces lean ground turkey breast

½ teaspoon extra-virgin olive oil

½ garlic clove, crushed

2 teaspoons finely chopped fresh parsley

½ teaspoon finely chopped fresh rosemary

Olive oil spray

⅓ of the roasted mixed veggies

4 cups chopped fresh spinach

¼ avocado, sliced

### DIRECTIONS

1. Using your hands as a tool, mix the turkey, olive oil, garlic, parsley, and rosemary together until well combined. Flatten into a patty.
2. Heat a medium skillet over medium-high heat and spray with olive oil. Cook the turkey patty for 6 minutes on each side. Set aside.
3. Place the roasted veggies in the pan to heat through. Add the spinach and stir into the veggies until wilted.
4. Place the turkey patty on the veggies and top with avocado.

### NUTRITIONAL INFORMATION PER SERVING

255 calories, 23g protein, 24g carbs, 7g fat, 6g fiber

## Herbed Turkey Meatball and Veggie Soup

### INGREDIENTS

Olive oil spray

¼ cup sliced celery

¼ cup chopped onion

1 garlic clove, crushed

1 sprig of fresh thyme

4 ounces lean ground turkey breast

1 cup chopped broccoli

1 cup shredded cabbage

2 cups low-sodium vegetable broth

1 tablespoon roughly chopped fresh parsley

1 cup chopped Swiss chard

### DIRECTIONS

1. Coat a medium saucepan with olive oil spray and heat over medium-high heat. Add the celery and onion and cook for 6 minutes. Stir in the garlic and thyme.
2. Form the turkey into little meatballs and add to the pot.
3. Cook the meatballs for 5 to 7 minutes, until browned, turning occasionally.
4. Add the broccoli, cabbage, and broth. Simmer for 20 minutes.
5. Turn off the heat, stir in the parsley and Swiss chard, and remove the thyme sprig.

### NUTRITIONAL INFORMATION PER SERVING

263 calories, 24g protein, 27g carbs, 5g fat, 7g fiber

## Chicken Alla Fresca

INGREDIENTS

1 teaspoon Dijon mustard

1 teaspoon red wine vinegar

Cracked black pepper

1 tomato, quartered

1 cup cubed watermelon

1 radish, thinly sliced

1 tablespoon chopped fresh basil

1 tablespoon chopped fresh parsley

2 tablespoons chopped celery leaves

¼ avocado, cubed

6 cups chopped mixed greens

4 ounces roasted chicken breast, cubed

DIRECTIONS

1. Whisk the Dijon, vinegar, and a sprinkle of pepper.
2. In a large bowl, gently toss all other ingredients with the dressing.

NUTRITIONAL INFORMATION PER SERVING

269 calories, 25g protein, 22g carbs, 8g fat, 3g fiber

## Jumbo Stir-Fry

### INGREDIENTS

Olive oil spray

½ teaspoon toasted light sesame oil

4 ounces skinless, boneless raw chicken, sliced

½ cup sliced celery

1 head of baby bok choy, chopped

1 cup chopped broccoli

1 cup chopped cauliflower

1 cup shredded cabbage

4 cups chopped fresh spinach

½ tablespoon Bragg's Liquid Aminos

2 tablespoons low-sodium vegetable broth

½ teaspoon crushed red pepper

### DIRECTIONS

1. Coat a large skillet with olive oil spray and sesame oil. Add the chicken and stir-fry for 3 minutes.

2. Add the celery, bok choy, broccoli, cauliflower, and cabbage and stir-fry for 4 minutes.

3. Add the spinach, Bragg's Aminos, broth, and crushed red pepper. Simmer until the veggies are fork-tender.

### NUTRITIONAL INFORMATION PER SERVING

245 calories, 30g protein, 13g carbs, 6g fat, 10g fiber

## Spaghetti Squash Bolognese

### INGREDIENTS
4 ounces lean ground turkey breast

¼ cup sliced celery

¼ yellow onion, finely chopped

½ cup Bob's marinara

1 cup spaghetti squash strands

3 cups chopped fresh spinach

### DIRECTIONS
1. Heat a medium saucepan over medium-high heat. Combine the turkey, celery, and onion in the pot.
2. Sauté for 8 minutes, stirring occasionally to break the turkey apart.
3. Add the marinara and simmer for 20 minutes. Mix in the spaghetti squash (which will warm through from the heat of the sauce).
4. Turn off the heat, add the spinach, and stir until wilted.

### NUTRITIONAL INFORMATION PER SERVING
273 calories, 22g protein, 25g carbs, 6g fat, 7g fiber

## Orange and Parsley Fish "Pockets" with Roasted Asparagus and Fennel

### INGREDIENTS

Olive oil spray

½ fennel bulb, thinly sliced

8 raw asparagus spears, trimmed and cut into 1½-inch pieces

1 tablespoon chopped fresh parsley leaves

4 ounces halibut or cod

1 tablespoon freshly squeezed orange juice

1 cup spaghetti squash strands

4 cups chopped arugula

### DIRECTIONS

1. Preheat the oven to 400°F. Place a 12-inch sheet of foil on a baking sheet. Coat with olive oil spray.
2. Toss the fennel, asparagus, and parsley and place on the foil. Top with the fish and drizzle orange juice on top.
3. Fold the foil over the fish and fennel/asparagus, folding and crimping the edges tightly to seal and enclose the filling completely.
4. Bake the fish "pockets" for 17 minutes.
5. During the last few minutes of baking, warm the spaghetti squash. Place on a plate with the arugula, then slide the contents of the packet on top.

### NUTRITIONAL INFORMATION PER SERVING

282 calories, 28g protein, 20g carbs, 7g fat, 9g fiber

## WEEK 2

*Prepare Ahead and Store*

## Whole-Wheat or Whole-Grain Penne Pasta

INGREDIENTS

⅔ cup whole-wheat or whole-grain penne pasta

Olive oil spray

DIRECTIONS

1. Bring water to a boil in a medium pot.
2. Add the pasta and cook 7 to 10 minutes, until al dente, stirring occasionally.
3. Drain and let cool.
4. Spray the pasta with olive oil to avoid sticking. Store the pasta in a plastic zip-top bag.

*Note: You will use this precooked pasta twice this week.*

NUTRITIONAL INFORMATION PER SERVING:

104 calories, 5g protein, 22g carbs, 2g fat, 2g fiber

## Roasted Mixed Vegetables

### INGREDIENTS

2 zucchini, cut into ½-inch pieces

2 yellow squash, cut into ½-inch pieces

12 large asparagus spears, each cut into four pieces

1 pint cherry tomatoes, halved

1 garlic clove, slivered

Olive oil spray

1 teaspoon dried thyme, herbes de Provence, or Italian seasoning

Cracked black pepper

### DIRECTIONS

1. Preheat the oven to 400°F.
2. Place the vegetables and garlic in a baking dish and coat evenly with a light spritz of olive oil.
3. Toss with the thyme and a sprinkle of pepper and roast for 20 minutes.
4. When cool, store in an airtight container in the fridge.

*Note: This recipe will be used in three meals during the week.*

### NUTRITIONAL INFORMATION PER SERVING

72 calories, 5g protein, 14g carbs, 1g fat, 5g fiber

## Roasted Chicken Breast

---

### INGREDIENTS

Olive oil spray

5 4-ounce skinless, boneless chicken breasts

Cracked black pepper

### DIRECTIONS

1. Preheat the oven to 350°F.
2. Spray a baking sheet with olive oil.
3. Lay the chicken breasts on the baking sheet in a single layer.
4. Coat lightly with olive oil spray and cracked pepper.
5. Bake for 15 to 20 minutes or until the juices run clear.

*Note: Each chicken breast will be used individually in meals during the week.*

### NUTRITIONAL INFORMATION PER SERVING

134 calories, 25g protein, 0g carbs, 3g fat, 0g fiber

## Roasted Cauliflower

### INGREDIENTS
2 heads of cauliflower
Olive oil spray
Cracked black pepper

### DIRECTIONS
1. Preheat the oven to 450°F. Bring a large pot of water to a boil.
2. Separate the cauliflower into large florets and plunge them into the boiling water for 3 minutes, or until cooked al dente.
3. Drain, pat dry with paper towel or clean dish cloth, and place in a single layer in a baking dish.
4. Spray with olive oil, then sprinkle with pepper to taste.
5. Roast for 10 to 15 minutes, until the tops begin to brown.

*Note: You will use this cauliflower in three recipes this week.*

### NUTRITIONAL INFORMATION PER SERVING
66 calories, 5g protein, 13g carbs, 1g fat, 5g fiber

## Roasted Tomatoes

INGREDIENTS

    6 plum tomatoes
    Olive oil spray
    Cracked black pepper (optional)

DIRECTIONS

1.  Preheat the oven to 450°F.
2.  Cut the tomatoes into quarters.
3.  Lay the tomatoes in a baking dish and coat with the olive oil spray and pepper (if desired).
4.  Cover with foil and bake for 1 hour 15 minutes.

*Note: Roasting the tomatoes at this heat and for this length of time will reduce them to an almost sun-dried state. You will use these tomatoes in two recipes this week.*

NUTRITIONAL INFORMATION PER SERVING:

    33 calories, 2g protein, 7g carbs, 0g fat, 2g fiber

# Roasted Asparagus

**INGREDIENTS**

8 asparagus spears

Olive oil spray

Cracked black pepper (optional)

**DIRECTIONS**

1. Preheat the oven to 425°F.
2. Place the asparagus on a baking sheet, coat evenly with a spritz of olive oil, sprinkle with pepper if desired, and toss. Rearrange the spears in a single layer.
3. Roast for 10 minutes.

*Note: You will use this asparagus in two recipes this week.*

**NUTRITIONAL INFORMATION PER SERVING:**

26 calories, 3g protein, 5g carbs, 0g fat, 3g fiber

## Arugula Pesto

INGREDIENTS

    2 cups roughly chopped arugula

    ¼ cup low-sodium vegetable broth

    1 garlic clove

    1 tablespoon fresh lemon juice

    2 tablespoons toasted walnuts or cashews

DIRECTIONS

    In a blender or food processor, process all ingredients until smooth.

*Note: This pesto will be used in two meals during the week.*

NUTRITIONAL INFORMATION PER SERVING

    68 calories, 2g protein, 3g carbs, 6g fat, 1g fiber

## CHOP AHEAD AND STORE

**Tropical fruit dice**

1 cup diced pineapple

1 cup diced mango

Note: You will use this diced fruit twice this week.

**3 or 4 large bunches of kale (yield 9 cups chopped)**

Remove the leaves from the stems and ribs and chop into
big pieces.

**1 large bunch of Swiss chard (yield 3 cups chopped)**

Remove the leaves from the stems and ribs and chop into big pieces.

**3 medium zucchini**

Cut into thin matchsticks.

**1 large head of broccoli**

Chop roughly.

*Week 2 Power Breakfasts*

## Scrambled Pasta

INGREDIENTS

    1 teaspoon olive oil

    3 cups chopped fresh spinach

    5 egg whites, lightly beaten

    ½ of the precooked penne

    2 tablespoons finely chopped fresh parsley

    ½ tablespoon grated Parmesan cheese

DIRECTIONS

1. Coat a pan with the olive oil and heat over medium heat.
2. Place the spinach in the pan and cook until wilted. Set aside on a paper towel to absorb the liquid.
3. Pour the egg whites into the pan and begin to scramble them.
4. After a minute, add the spinach, pasta, parsley, and Parmesan.
5. Mix until the eggs are cooked through and the pasta is warm.

NUTRITIONAL INFORMATION PER SERVING

    264 calories, 26g protein, 27g carbs, 6g fat, 6g fiber

# Turkey Scramble

### INGREDIENTS

Olive oil spray

1 3-inch sweet potato

1 cup chopped red bell pepper

2 ounces lean ground turkey breast

½ tablespoon chopped fresh cilantro

3 egg whites, lightly beaten

Cracked black pepper

### DIRECTIONS

1. Puncture the sweet potato several times with a fork. Microwave 10 to 15 minutes, until tender. To be served on the side.
2. Coat a pan with olive oil spray and heat over medium-high heat.
3. Add the bell pepper to the pan and sauté for 5 minutes, stirring occasionally.
4. Add the turkey and cook for about 7 minutes, stirring occasionally to break up the meat, until browned.
5. Mix in the cilantro, egg whites, and spinach. Sprinkle with pepper.
6. Scramble until the eggs are cooked through.

### NUTRITIONAL INFORMATION PER SERVING

285 calories, 30g protein, 21g carbs, 6g fat, 7g fiber

## Yogurt with Tropical Fruit

INGREDIENTS

　　1 cup nonfat Greek yogurt
　　1 cup diced tropical fruit mixture
　　1½ tablespoons ground flaxseed

DIRECTIONS

　　Place the yogurt in a bowl, top with the fruit, and sprinkle with
　　the flaxseed.

NUTRITIONAL INFORMATION PER SERVING

　　264 calories, 20g protein, 27g carbs, 3g fat, 3g fiber

## Spicy Asparagus and Quinoa

INGREDIENTS

½ cup water

¼ cup quinoa

¼ cup nonfat Greek yogurt

1 teaspoon Dijon mustard

½ teaspoon hot sauce

1 teaspoon fresh lemon juice

8 roasted asparagus spears, cut into 1-inch pieces

½ tablespoon chopped toasted cashews or walnuts

DIRECTIONS

1. Bring the water to a boil in a small saucepan.
2. Add the quinoa to the boiling water, stir, and reduce the heat to low.
3. Cover and let simmer until cooked and fluffy, about 15 minutes.
4. Let sit for 5 minutes, then fluff with a fork.
5. In a small bowl, whisk the yogurt, Dijon, hot sauce, and lemon juice.
6. In your breakfast bowl, toss the asparagus, cooked quinoa, and nuts.
7. Drizzle the yogurt mixture on top of the quinoa mixture.

NUTRITIONAL INFORMATION PER SERVING

267 calories, 24g protein, 23g carbs, 7g fat, 6g fiber

## Pasta with Pesto Eggs

INGREDIENTS

Olive oil spray

3 cups chopped fresh spinach

5 egg whites, lightly beaten

½ of the precooked penne

½ cup arugula pesto

DIRECTIONS

1. Coat a medium skillet with olive oil spray and set over medium heat.
2. Place the spinach in the pan and cook until wilted. Set aside on a paper towel to absorb the liquid.
3. Pour the egg whites into the pan and begin to scramble them.
4. After a minute, add the pasta, spinach, and pesto.
5. Mix until the eggs are cooked through and the pasta is warm.

NUTRITIONAL INFORMATION PER SERVING:

278 calories, 27g protein, 24g carbs, 7g fat, 6g fiber

## Applesauce Oatmeal with a Side of Green Eggs

### INGREDIENTS
⅓ cup rolled oats
⅓ cup natural unsweetened applesauce
½ teaspoon ground cinnamon
½ teaspoon vanilla extract
3 cups chopped fresh spinach
4 egg whites, lightly beaten

### DIRECTIONS
1. In a small pot, combine the oats, applesauce, cinnamon, and vanilla. Bring to a simmer and cook until done, about 5 minutes.
2. Heat a skillet over medium heat and spray with olive oil. Add the spinach and cook until wilted. Set aside on a paper towel to absorb the liquid.
3. Pour the egg whites into the hot pan, then add the spinach and scramble until cooked through.

### NUTRITIONAL INFORMATION PER SERVING
255 calories, 25g protein, 26g carbs, 5g fat, 3g fiber

## Cucumber-Blueberry Shake with a Side of Eggs

INGREDIENTS

2 Persian cucumbers, cut into 1-inch pieces

½ cup blueberries

2 cups chopped dandelion greens

1 cup unsweetened almond milk

1 tablespoon ground flaxseed

Olive oil spray

4 egg whites, lightly beaten

Cracked black pepper

DIRECTIONS

1. In a blender, blend the cucumbers, blueberries, dandelion greens, almond milk, and flaxseed.
2. Heat a skillet over medium-high heat and spray with olive oil.
3. Add the egg whites to the pan, sprinkle with black pepper, and scramble until cooked through.
4. Sip your shake with a smile while eating your scrambled egg whites.

NUTRITIONAL INFORMATION PER SERVING

277 calories, 23g protein, 26g carbs, 8g fat, 8g fiber

## Week 2 Lean Lunches

## Kale Salad

### INGREDIENTS

> 2 tablespoons chopped green onions (scallions), both white and
> green parts
> ½ tablespoon apple cider vinegar
> 1 tablespoon fresh lemon juice
> 2 cups chopped kale
> 4 ounces roasted chicken breast, shredded
> ¼ avocado, cubed
> 5 cups chopped mixed greens
> ¼ apple, cubed
> ½ cup chopped broccoli

### DIRECTIONS

1. In a small bowl, whisk the green onions, vinegar, and lemon juice.
2. Put the kale in a large bowl and massage the dressing into it.
3. Toss with the chicken, avocado, mixed greens, apple, and broccoli.

### NUTRITIONAL INFORMATION PER SERVING

280 calories, 27g protein, 22g carbs, 9g fat, 5g fiber

## Roasted Tomato Salad

INGREDIENTS

1 cup roasted tomatoes

1 tablespoon toasted cashews or walnuts

½ tablespoon drained and rinsed capers

6 cups chopped mixed greens

3 Persian cucumbers, diced

½ cup diced red bell pepper

1 teaspoon minced fresh chives

4 ounces roasted chicken breast, shredded

Cracked black pepper

DIRECTIONS

Lightly toss all ingredients in your favorite salad bowl.

NUTRITIONAL INFORMATION PER SERVING

275 calories, 27g protein, 24g carbs, 6g fat, 7g fiber

## Roasted Vegetable Salad with Turkey

INGREDIENTS

1 tablespoon balsamic vinegar

1 teaspoon extra-virgin olive oil

1 teaspoon Dijon mustard

Cracked black pepper

⅓ of the roasted mixed vegetables

2 cups chopped arugula

4 cups chopped mixed greens

4 ounces no-salt sliced turkey breast

DIRECTIONS

1. In a small bowl, whisk the balsamic, olive oil, Dijon, and cracked pepper.
2. Lightly toss the dressing with the roasted vegetables, arugula, mixed greens, and turkey.

NUTRITIONAL INFORMATION PER SERVING

270 calories, 24g protein, 21g carbs, 6g fat, 6g fiber

## Pesto Chicken Salad

INGREDIENTS

¼ cup arugula pesto

4 ounces roasted chicken breast, shredded

½ cup chopped zucchini

2 Persian cucumbers, chopped

1 plum tomato, sliced

½ cup chopped red bell pepper

2 leaves of butter leaf lettuce

DIRECTIONS

1. In a medium bowl, mix the pesto with the chicken.
2. Toss with the remaining ingredients.

NUTRITIONAL INFORMATION PER SERVING

276 calories, 26g protein, 19g carbs, 6g fat, 5g fiber

## Chopped Salad

INGREDIENTS
    2 teaspoons balsamic vinegar
    ¾ teaspoon extra-virgin olive oil
    1 tablespoon finely chopped fresh parsley
    ½ teaspoon finely chopped garlic
    5 ounces no-salt sliced turkey breast
    6 cups chopped mixed greens
    2 Persian cucumbers, chopped
    ½ cup chopped red bell pepper
    1 plum tomato, chopped

DIRECTIONS
    1.  In a small bowl, whisk the balsamic, olive oil, parsley, and
        garlic.
    2.  Lightly toss with the turkey, greens, cucumbers, red pepper,
        and tomato.

NUTRITIONAL INFORMATION PER SERVING
    279 calories, 25g protein, 25g carbs, 6g fat, 4g fiber

## Buffalo Chicken Salad

INGREDIENTS

4 ounces roasted chicken breast, shredded

½ teaspoon extra-virgin olive oil

1 teaspoon hot sauce

2 tablespoons nonfat Greek yogurt

2 Persian cucumbers, chopped

1 cup chopped red bell pepper

6 cups chopped mixed greens

DIRECTIONS

1. In a medium bowl, blend the olive oil, hot sauce, and yogurt. Mix in the chicken.

2. Lightly toss with the remaining ingredients.

NUTRITIONAL INFORMATION PER SERVING

260 calories, 28g protein, 22g carbs, 6g fat, 4g fiber

# Taco Salad

## INGREDIENTS

5 ounces lean ground turkey breast
1 plum tomato, chopped
3 cups chopped spinach
1 cup roasted cauliflower
1 tablespoon chopped fresh cilantro
1 tablespoon nonfat plain Greek yogurt
1 tablespoon chopped green onion (scallion)
Pinch of cayenne
Cracked pepper

## DIRECTIONS

1. Cook the ground turkey until browned in a medium skillet. Remove from heat.
2. Add tomatoes and cilantro to the skillet and season the mixture with cracked pepper and cayenne.
3. Spoon turkey and tomato mixture over the spinach and garnish with yogurt and green onion
4. Serve cauliflower on the side.

## NUTRITIONAL INFORMATION PER SERVING

249 calories, 28g protein, 13g carbs, 6g fat, 5g fiber

*Week 2 Thinner Dinners*

## Halibut "Tacos" with Tropical Salsa

### INGREDIENTS

Olive oil spray

4 ounces halibut (or cod)

1 teaspoon extra-virgin olive oil

Cracked black pepper (optional)

1 cup diced tropical fruit

1 tablespoon finely chopped green onion (scallion)

1 tablespoon finely chopped fresh cilantro

½ tablespoon fresh lime juice

½ cup chopped zucchini

2 cups chopped fresh spinach

2 leaves of butter leaf lettuce

### DIRECTIONS

1. Preheat the oven to 400°F.
2. Spray a baking sheet lightly with olive oil. Place the fish on the baking sheet and top with 1 teaspoon extra-virgin olive oil. Sprinkle with pepper, if desired, and bake for 15 minutes.
3. Meanwhile, combine the tropical fruit, green onion, cilantro, lime, and zucchini.
4. Place 1 cup spinach in each lettuce leaf. Top each with half the fish and some tropical salsa.

### NUTRITIONAL INFORMATION PER SERVING

260 calories, 25g protein, 23g carbs, 7g fat, 3g fiber

## Green Cauliflower Soup

### INGREDIENTS

2 cups roasted cauliflower

1 cup low-sodium vegetable broth

1 tablespoon chopped fresh dill

2 cups roughly chopped fresh spinach

Cracked black pepper (optional)

4 ounces roasted chicken breast, shredded

1 cup chopped red bell pepper

### DIRECTIONS

1. Combine the cauliflower, broth, dill, and spinach in a medium saucepan and bring to a simmer. Add black pepper if desired and simmer for 5 minutes.
2. Let cool slightly, then pour into a blender and puree until smooth.
3. Pour back into the pot, add the chicken and bell pepper, and simmer for 10 minutes.

### NUTRITIONAL INFORMATION PER SERVING

257 calories, 27g protein, 22g carbs, 5g fat, 7g fiber

## Shrimp Skimpy

### INGREDIENTS

1 garlic clove, slivered

1 teaspoon extra-virgin olive oil

1 cup chopped broccoli

½ cup low-sodium vegetable broth

Pinch of crushed red pepper

Freshly ground black pepper to taste

1 tablespoon fresh lemon juice

5 ounces shrimp, peeled and deveined

1 tablespoon finely chopped fresh parsley

3 cups chopped Swiss chard

*Side Salad*

5 cups chopped mixed greens

1 cup chopped red bell pepper

2 Persian cucumbers, chopped

2 teaspoons balsamic vinegar

1 tablespoon fresh lemon juice

### DIRECTIONS

1. In a medium skillet, warm the garlic and olive oil over medium-low heat for 2 minutes.
2. Add the broccoli and increase the heat to medium-high. Stir and sauté for 4 minutes.
3. Add the broth, crushed red pepper, black pepper, and lemon juice and bring to a simmer.
4. Add the shrimp and cook until pink, approximately 5 minutes.

5. Throw in the parsley and Swiss chard and stir until just wilted.
6. Toss the side salad ingredients together.

NUTRITIONAL INFORMATION PER SERVING

277 calories, 27g protein, 23g carbs, 7g fat, 7g fiber

## Steak and Pesto "Potatoes" with Roasted Asparagus

INGREDIENTS

Olive oil spray

5 ounces lean steak

Cracked black pepper

¼ cup low-sodium vegetable broth

2 cups roasted cauliflower

¼ cup arugula pesto

⅓ of the roasted asparagus

DIRECTIONS

1. Spray a medium skillet with olive oil and heat over medium-high heat.
2. Season the steak with cracked pepper and place in the pan. Cook 8 to 10 minutes on each side.
3. Meanwhile, in a small saucepan, heat the vegetable broth and cauliflower until simmering.
4. Carefully transfer the hot contents from the saucepan into a blender, add the pesto, and puree until smooth.
5. Remove the steak and let rest on a plate.
6. Warm the roasted asparagus in the same pan as the steak.
7. Serve the steak with mashed "potatoes" and roasted veggies.

NUTRITIONAL INFORMATION PER SERVING

255 calories, 31g protein, 26g carbs, 5g fat, 6g fiber

## Mango Chicken

INGREDIENTS

Olive oil spray

4 ounces skinless, boneless raw chicken, sliced

1 cup chopped broccoli

1 cup chopped zucchini

½ tablespoon Bragg's Liquid Aminos

1 teaspoon rice vinegar

¼ cup low-sodium vegetable broth

¼ cup roughly chopped mango

3 cups chopped kale

DIRECTIONS

1. Lightly coat a medium skillet with olive oil spray, heat over medium-high heat, and add the chicken. Cook for 4 minutes, stirring occasionally.
2. Add the broccoli and zucchini. Sauté for 5 more minutes.
3. Drizzle in the Bragg's Aminos, rice vinegar, and broth and bring to a simmer.
4. Add the mango and kale and cook until the kale is slightly wilted.

NUTRITIONAL INFORMATION PER SERVING

255 calories, 28g protein, 25g carbs, 4g fat, 6g fiber

## Eggplant Chili

INGREDIENTS

1 teaspoon olive oil

1 garlic clove, crushed

1 cup diced eggplant

4 ounces lean ground turkey breast

1 cup roasted tomatoes

1 cup low-sodium vegetable broth

3 cups finely chopped fresh spinach

Cracked black pepper (optional)

1 tablespoon chopped fresh cilantro

DIRECTIONS

1. Heat the olive oil in a medium pot over medium-high heat. Add the garlic and eggplant and cook for 5 minutes.

2. Add the turkey and cook for about 7 minutes, stirring occasionally to break up the meat, until browned.

3. Add the tomatoes and broth and simmer for 20 minutes.

4. Add the spinach and cook until just wilted.

5. Turn off the heat, add black pepper if desired, stir in the cilantro, and serve.

NUTRITIONAL INFORMATION PER SERVING

279 calories, 24g protein, 23g carbs, 7g fat, 7g fiber

# Spicy Roasted Chicken with Veggies

## INGREDIENTS

4 ounces raw chicken, cubed

1 cup chopped broccoli

1 cup sliced zucchini, cut into ½-inch circles

1 cup chopped cauliflower

1 cup sliced yellow squash, cut into ½-inch circles

1 small garlic clove, slivered

Pinch of crushed red pepper

1 teaspoon chopped fresh thyme

Olive oil spray

*Side Salad*

5 cups mixed greens

2 Persian cucumbers, chopped

2 teaspoons balsamic vinegar

1 tablespoon fresh lemon juice

## DIRECTIONS

1. Preheat the oven to 425°F.
2. Place the chicken, vegetables, and seasonings in a glass baking dish. Coat with olive oil spray and mix.
3. Bake for 15 minutes.
4. Toss the side salad ingredients together.

## NUTRITIONAL INFORMATION PER SERVING

260 calories, 27g protein, 16g carbs, 8g fat, 6g fiber

# WEEK 3

*Prepare Ahead and Store*

## Ratatouille

### INGREDIENTS

    1 large eggplant

    2 zucchini

    3 tomatoes

    1 red bell pepper

    Olive oil spray

    1 garlic clove, thinly sliced

    1 tablespoon balsamic vinegar

    Cracked black pepper (optional)

    2 teaspoons chopped fresh thyme

### DIRECTIONS

1. Preheat the oven to 400°F.
2. Cut all vegetables into ⅓-inch dice and place in a baking dish. Coat evenly with a light spritz of olive oil.
3. Toss the chopped veggies with the garlic and balsamic vinegar; sprinkle with pepper if desired.
4. Roast for 30 minutes.
5. When done, mix in the thyme.

*Note: This recipe will be used in three meals during the week.*

### NUTRITIONAL INFORMATION PER SERVING

    103 calories, 4g protein, 32g carbs, 1g fat, 8g fiber

## Cooked Quinoa

INGREDIENTS

1 cup water

½ cup quinoa

DIRECTIONS

1. Bring the water to a boil in a small saucepan.
2. Add the quinoa to the boiling water, stir, and reduce the heat to low.
3. Cover and let simmer until cooked and fluffy, about 15 minutes. Turn off heat.
4. Let sit for 5 minutes, then fluff with a fork.

*Note: This will be used in two breakfast recipes.*

NUTRITIONAL INFORMATION PER SERVING

156 calories, 6g protein, 27g carbs, 3g fat, 3g fiber

## Red Cabbage Slaw

INGREDIENTS

3 cups shredded red cabbage

2 tablespoons red wine vinegar

½ tablespoon chopped fresh oregano

1 tablespoon orange juice

DIRECTIONS

Lightly toss all ingredients and store in an airtight container in the fridge.

*Note: This will be used in two meals during the week.*

NUTRITIONAL INFORMATION PER SERVING

46 calories, 2g protein, 11g carbs, 0g fat, 3g fiber

## Roasted Chicken Breast

INGREDIENTS

Olive oil spray

4 4-ounce skinless, boneless chicken breasts

Cracked black pepper

DIRECTIONS

1. Preheat the oven to 350°F.
2. Spray a baking sheet with olive oil.
3. Lay the chicken breasts on the baking sheet in a single layer.
4. Coat lightly with olive oil spray and cracked pepper.
5. Bake for 15 to 20 minutes or until the juices run clear.

*Note: This will be used in four meals during the week.*

NUTRITIONAL INFORMATION PER SERVING:

134 calories, 25g protein, 0g carbs, 3g fat, 0g fiber

## Roasted Asparagus

### INGREDIENTS
16 asparagus spears

Olive oil spray

Cracked black pepper (optional)

### DIRECTIONS
1. Preheat the oven to 425°F.
2. Spread the asparagus on a baking sheet, coat evenly with a spritz of olive oil, sprinkle with black pepper if desired, and toss. Rearrange the asparagus in a single layer.
3. Roast for 10 minutes.

*Note: This will be used in two meals during the week.*

### NUTRITIONAL INFORMATION PER SERVING::
26 calories, 3g protein, 5g carbs, 0g fat, 3g fiber

---

**CUT CHOP AHEAD AND STORE**

1 or 2 large bunches of kale (yield 5 cups chopped)

Remove leaves from stems and ribs, then chop into big pieces.

1 large bunch of Swiss chard (yield 3 cups chopped)

Remove leaves from stems and ribs, then chop into big pieces.

## *Week 3 Power Breakfasts*

## Ratatouille Scramble

### INGREDIENTS
Olive oil spray
⅓ of the ratatouille
5 egg whites, lightly beaten
½ slice of Ezekiel bread

### DIRECTIONS
1. Lightly coat a medium skillet with olive oil spray and heat over medium-high heat. Add the ratatouille and warm through for 2 minutes.
2. Lower the heat to medium and add the egg whites. Scramble until the eggs are cooked, approximately 5 minutes.
3. Toast the Ezekiel bread and serve with the eggs.

### NUTRITIONAL INFORMATION PER SERVING
269 calories, 26g protein, 28g carbs, 7g fat, 11g fiber

## Spanish Scramble

### INGREDIENTS

1 teaspoon extra-virgin olive oil
¼ cup peeled and thin-sliced sweet potato
½ red bell pepper, thinly sliced
¼ medium onion, thinly sliced
5 egg whites
¼ cup chopped fresh parsley
3 cups finely chopped fresh spinach
½ teaspoon hot sauce

### DIRECTIONS

1. Preheat the oven to 375°F.
2. Coat a medium ovenproof skillet with olive oil and heat over medium heat.
3. Add the potato, bell pepper, and onion. Cover and cook, stirring occasionally, until the potato is crisp-tender, 14 to 16 minutes. Uncover and cook for 1 to 2 more minutes.
4. In a bowl, whisk the egg whites, parsley, spinach, and hot sauce. Pour the egg mixture over the vegetables and stir to distribute evenly.
5. Bake for 12 to 16 minutes, or until whites are set and the top is lightly browned.

### NUTRITIONAL INFORMATION PER SERVING

275 calories, 24g protein, 27g carbs, 6g fat, 7g fiber

## Sweet Potato Hash

INGREDIENTS

½ sweet potato, cut into ¼-inch dice

½ green pepper, chopped

½ garlic clove, crushed

2 cups chopped kale

5 egg whites

1 green onion (scallion), chopped

1 tablespoon chopped fresh parsley

DIRECTIONS

1. Coat a medium skillet with olive oil spray and heat over medium heat.
2. Add the potato, green pepper, and garlic. Cover and cook, stirring occasionally, until the potato is crisp-tender, 14 to 16 minutes.
3. Uncover, add the kale, and cook for another 3 to 4 minutes, or until the kale is wilted.
4. Meanwhile, in a small bowl, whisk the egg whites with the green onion and parsley.
5. Add the eggs to the vegetables, scramble, and cook through. Or, plate the potato, then scramble the egg mixture in the same pan and serve next to the potato.

NUTRITIONAL INFORMATION PER SERVING

260 calories, 23g protein, 24g carbs, 6g fat, 6g fiber

## Stuffed Tomato

INGREDIENTS

1 large beefsteak tomato

5 egg whites

½ teaspoon finely chopped fresh chives

1 teaspoon finely chopped fresh parsley

½ tablespoon grated Parmesan cheese

DIRECTIONS

1. Preheat the oven to 350°F. Cut the top off the tomato and spoon out the flesh and seeds, discarding them. Be patient and try not to break the tomato.
2. Place the tomato in a small glass baking dish.
3. In a small bowl, whisk the egg whites with the chives and parsley.
4. Pour into the tomato and sprinkle on the Parmesan cheese. Bake until the egg mixture is set, 45 to 50 minutes. Serve warm.

NUTRITIONAL INFORMATION PER SERVING

264 calories, 26g protein, 28g carbs, 3g fat, 7g fiber

## Quinoaquiles

### INGREDIENTS

Olive oil spray

½ cup cooked quinoa

3 cups chopped fresh spinach

5 egg whites, lightly beaten

Cracked black pepper

1 tablespoon chopped fresh cilantro

1 teaspoon fresh lemon juice

1 teaspoon fresh lime juice

¼ avocado

### DIRECTIONS

1. Lightly coat a pan with olive oil spray and heat over medium-high heat. Add the quinoa, spinach, and egg whites and cook until the eggs are scrambled, 4 to 5 minutes. Add black pepper if desired.

2. In a small bowl, mash the cilantro, lemon, and lime with the avocado; sprinkle with pepper. Serve on top of the quinoaquiles.

### NUTRITIONAL INFORMATION PER SERVING

274 calories, 25g protein, 23g carbs, 7g fat, 5g fiber

## Shrimp and "Grits"

### INGREDIENTS

4 ounces shrimp, peeled and deveined

½ teaspoon Cajun seasoning, or to taste

2 tablespoons water

1 tablespoon sliced green onion (scallion)

1 cup chopped Swiss chard

¼ cup nonfat plain Greek yogurt

½ cup cooked quinoa, warmed

### DIRECTIONS

1. Lightly coat a small skillet with olive oil spray and heat over medium-high heat. Add the shrimp and Cajun seasoning and cook for 3 minutes on each side.
2. Add the water, green onion, and Swiss chard and cook, stirring, until the chard is wilted.
3. Stir in the Greek yogurt and serve on top of warm quinoa.

### NUTRITIONAL INFORMATION PER SERVING

277 calories, 25g protein, 21g carbs, 9g fat, 3g fiber

## Oatsotto

---

### INGREDIENTS

Olive oil spray

½ onion, chopped

6 cremini mushrooms, finely chopped

Cracked black pepper

½ cup rolled oats

1 cup low-sodium vegetable broth

2 cups chopped fresh spinach

5 egg whites, lightly beaten

### DIRECTIONS

1. Lightly coat a saucepan with olive oil spray and heat over medium-high heat. Add the onion and mushrooms. Cook for 6 minutes, stirring once.
2. Add the cracked pepper and oats. Cook for 2 more minutes. Pour in the broth and stir until the oats are cooked, about 5 minutes.
3. Turn off the heat and stir in the spinach. Remove from saucepan.
4. Scramble the egg whites in saucepan and then place the scrambled whites on top of the oat and spinach mixture.

### NUTRITIONAL INFORMATION PER SERVING

260 calories, 26g protein, 24g carbs, 6g fat, 2g fiber

*Week 3 Lean Lunches*

## Not-So-FAToosh

### INGREDIENTS

4 ounces roasted chicken breast, cubed

2 tablespoons nonfat plain Greek yogurt

1 plum tomato, chopped

1 radish, thinly sliced

1 Persian cucumber, chopped

1 cup chopped green bell pepper

5 cups chopped mixed greens

1 green onion (scallion), thinly sliced

1 tablespoon chopped fresh mint

2 tablespoons coarsely chopped fresh parsley

½ garlic clove, crushed

½ tablespoon fresh lemon juice

1 teaspoon extra-virgin olive oil

1 teaspoon cider or white wine vinegar

Cracked black pepper

### DIRECTIONS

1. In your favorite salad bowl, combine the chicken, yogurt, tomato, radish, cucumber, and bell pepper.
2. In a separate bowl, whisk the green onion, mint, parsley, garlic, lemon juice, olive oil, vinegar, and black pepper.
3. Toss the salad lightly with the dressing.

### NUTRITIONAL INFORMATION PER SERVING

241 calories, 26g protein, 12g carbs, 8g fat, 5g fiber

## Gazpacho Shrimp Salad

INGREDIENTS

5 ounces large shrimp, cooked and peeled

2 Persian cucumbers, chopped

1 plum tomato, diced

1 cup chopped red bell pepper

6 cups chopped mixed greens

1 green onion (scallion), sliced diagonally

1 tablespoon finely chopped fresh parsley

½ teaspoon chopped fresh chives

½ tablespoon red wine vinegar

1 teaspoon olive oil

⅛ teaspoon hot sauce

½ garlic clove, crushed

DIRECTIONS

1. Toss the shrimp, cucumber, tomato, bell pepper, and mixed greens together.
2. In a separate bowl, whisk the green onion, parsley, chives, vinegar, olive oil, hot sauce, and garlic.
3. Toss the salad lightly with the dressing.

NUTRITIONAL INFORMATION PER SERVING

264 calories, 27g protein, 18g carbs, 7g fat, 8g fiber

## Chicken Cucumber Salad

INGREDIENTS

1 tablespoon fresh lemon juice

1 tablespoon finely chopped fresh parsley

1 tablespoon finely chopped fresh basil

1 teaspoon drained, rinsed, and chopped capers

8 roasted asparagus spears, cut into 1-inch pieces

½ cup chopped red bell pepper

4 ounces roasted chicken breast, shredded

1 Persian cucumber, sliced

½ avocado, sliced

3 cups chopped fresh spinach

3 cups chopped mixed greens

Cracked black pepper

DIRECTIONS

Combine all ingredients with laughter and joy.

NUTRITIONAL INFORMATION PER SERVING

262 calories, 27g protein, 15g carbs, 8g fat, 7g fiber

# Ratatouille Salad

## INGREDIENTS
⅓ of the ratatouille
4 ounces roasted chicken breast, cubed
2 cups chopped arugula
1 tablespoon fresh lemon juice
1 teaspoon Dijon mustard
½ tablespoon balsamic vinegar

## DIRECTIONS
1. Place the ratatouille, chicken, and arugula in a bowl.
2. Whisk the lemon juice, Dijon, and balsamic together, pour over the salad, and toss.

## NUTRITIONAL INFORMATION PER SERVING
269 calories, 27g protein, 24g carbs, 8g fat, 9g fiber

## Red Cabbage Slaw with Steak

INGREDIENTS

4 ounces lean steak, cooked and sliced

8 spears roasted asparagus

1½ cups red cabbage slaw

Cracked black pepper

¼ avocado, sliced

DIRECTIONS

1. Heat the steak and asparagus.
2. Place on top of the prepared slaw along with a dash of pepper and the sliced avocado.

NUTRITIONAL INFORMATION PER SERVING

173 calories, 29g protein, 15g carbs, 6g fat, 10g fiber

# Jolly Green Salmon

### INGREDIENTS

1 tablespoon fresh lemon juice

1 tablespoon grated Parmesan cheese

1 teaspoon Dijon mustard

4 ounces salmon

Olive oil spray

8 raw asparagus spears

2 cups chopped zucchini

1 plum tomato, sliced

### DIRECTIONS

1. Preheat the oven to 400°F.
2. Mix the lemon, Parmesan, and Dijon in a small bowl. Coat the salmon with the mixture.
3. Lightly coat a baking sheet with olive oil spray. Lay the asparagus in a single layer and top with the zucchini, the tomato, then the salmon.
4. Bake for 15 minutes.

### NUTRITIONAL INFORMATION PER SERVING

241 calories, 27g protein, 12g carbs, 7g fat, 7g fiber

## Confetti Salad

INGREDIENTS

4 ounces pork tenderloin or chop (remove all fat), cooked and sliced

1½ cups red cabbage slaw

1 cup chopped bell pepper

1 Persian cucumber, diced

6 cups chopped mixed greens

1 tablespoon chopped fresh cilantro

1 teaspoon almond butter

1 tablespoon water

½ tablespoon Bragg's Liquid Aminos

DIRECTIONS

1. Lightly toss the pork with the slaw, bell pepper, cucumber, and mixed greens.
2. In a small bowl, combine the cilantro, almond butter, water, and Bragg's Aminos.
3. Lightly toss with the salad.

NUTRITIONAL INFORMATION PER SERVING

250 calories, 26g protein, 13g carbs, 7g fat, 7g fiber

*Week 3 Thinner Dinners*

## Chicken Ratatouille

### INGREDIENTS
1 teaspoon extra-virgin olive oil
⅓ of the ratatouille
4 ounces roasted chicken breast, shredded

### DIRECTIONS
Combine all the ingredients in a small pot and heat through.

### NUTRITIONAL INFORMATION PER SERVING
250 calories, 24g protein, 24g carbs, 7g fat, 8g fiber

## Gourmet Pork "Chop"

### INGREDIENTS

½ teaspoon extra-virgin olive oil

4 ounces pork tenderloin

¼ onion, sliced

1 cup chopped zucchini

¼ cup low-sodium vegetable broth

1 teaspoon chopped fresh thyme

2 cups chopped kale

### DIRECTIONS

1. Drizzle the olive oil into a skillet and heat over medium-high heat. Add the pork and sear for 4 minutes on each side.
2. Transfer the pork to a plate. Add the onion and zucchini to the pan and sauté for 3 minutes. Pour in the broth and thyme and bring to a simmer.
3. Place the pork back in the pan, along with the kale. Cover and cook for 3 minutes, until the kale is wilted.

### NUTRITIONAL INFORMATION PER SERVING

258 calories, 29g protein, 19g carbs, 7g fat, 6g fiber

## Mediterranean Salad

INGREDIENTS

4 ounces low-sodium water-packed canned tuna

1 teaspoon red wine vinegar

1 teaspoon olive oil

2 teaspoons Dijon mustard

2 teaspoons drained and rinsed capers

2 Persian cucumbers, chopped

1 red bell pepper, chopped

2 plum tomatoes, chopped

4 cups chopped arugula

DIRECTIONS

1. Mix the tuna with the vinegar, olive oil, Dijon, and capers.

2. Lightly toss with the cucumbers, bell pepper, tomatoes, and arugula.

NUTRITIONAL INFORMATION PER SERVING

250 calories, 26g protein, 13g carbs, 8g fat, 7g fiber

## Chicken and Zucchini Pouch

### INGREDIENTS

1 teaspoon extra-virgin olive oil
1 cup chopped Broccolini
2 cups ½-inch sliced zucchini
2 teaspoons fresh lemon juice
1 teaspoon chopped fresh dill
Crushed red pepper
4 ounces boneless, skinless raw chicken breast
2 cups chopped fresh spinach

### DIRECTIONS

1. Preheat the oven to 350°F. Place a 12-inch sheet of foil on a baking sheet. Coat with the olive oil.
2. Toss the Broccolini and zucchini with 1 teaspoon of the lemon juice, the dill, and crushed red pepper. Place on the foil.
3. Top with the chicken and drizzle with the remaining 1 teaspoon lemon juice.
4. Fold the foil over the chicken and vegetables, folding and crimping the edges tightly to seal and enclose the filling completely.
5. Bake the packet for 20 minutes. Slide the contents onto a plate and serve with a spinach salad on the side (dressed lightly with lemon juice and balsamic vinegar).

### NUTRITIONAL INFORMATION PER SERVING

260 calories, 30g protein, 13g carbs, 8g fat, 7g fiber

## Herbed Chicken with Red Pepper

### INGREDIENTS

4 ounces boneless, skinless raw chicken breast

1 teaspoon each fresh parsley, oregano, and marjoram, chopped

½ garlic clove, thinly sliced

Pinch of crushed red pepper

4 stalks of Broccolini, each cut into four pieces

12 green beans

1 cup chopped red bell pepper

1 teaspoon extra-virgin olive oil

### DIRECTIONS

1. Preheat the oven to 425°F.
2. Place all ingredients in a glass baking dish and toss with the olive oil.
3. Bake for 15 minutes.

### NUTRITIONAL INFORMATION PER SERVING

261 calories, 27g protein, 16g carbs, 8g fat, 7g fiber

## Swiss Chard and Cabbage Stir-Fry

INGREDIENTS

1 teaspoon extra-virgin olive oil

¼ cup onion, finely chopped

½ garlic clove, crushed

½ cup low-sodium vegetable broth

4 ounces boneless, skinless raw chicken, cubed

1 cup shredded red cabbage

2 cups chopped Swiss chard

DIRECTIONS

1. Pour the olive oil into a medium skillet over medium-high heat. Add the onion and cook until translucent, approximately 5 minutes. Add the garlic and stir.
2. Add the broth and chicken and bring to a simmer. Cook for 8 to 10 minutes or until the chicken is no longer pink.
3. Add the cabbage and Swiss chard and cook for 3 more minutes, stirring occasionally, until wilted.

NUTRITIONAL INFORMATION PER SERVING

263 calories, 25g protein, 19g carbs, 8g fat, 7g fiber

## Gourmet Turkey Burger

### INGREDIENTS

4 ounces lean ground turkey breast
½ garlic clove, minced
2 teaspoons finely chopped fresh parsley
½ teaspoon finely chopped fresh rosemary
Olive oil spray
3 cups chopped mixed greens
2 teaspoons Dijon mustard
¼ avocado, sliced
1 tomato, sliced
2 cups chopped broccoli, steamed until just tender

### DIRECTIONS

1. Using your hands as a tool, mix the turkey, garlic, parsley, and rosemary together until well combined. Flatten into a patty.
2. Heat a small skillet and spray with olive oil. Cook the turkey patty for 6 minutes on each side.
3. Place on a bed of greens and top with Dijon, avocado, and tomato. Serve with steamed broccoli.

### NUTRITIONAL INFORMATION PER SERVING

273 calories, 23g protein, 22g carbs, 8g fat, 6g fiber

# THE END?

## TRANSITIONING TO *THE SKINNY RULES*

The honeymoon! The reunion! That long stretch of beach and all those coconuts . . . ahhh! Now it's time to stop all the deprivation, right?

Yes and no. I'm not going to spoil your fun. If you undertook the program in *Jumpstart to Skinny* in order to look fabulous for a specific event, then enjoy the event and the immediate aftermath. Celebrate the occasion!

But "immediate aftermath" doesn't mean the rest of the season. And it definitely shouldn't mean fast food, sugar binging, and processed or packaged crap!

Remember, *Jumpstart to Skinny* is a short-term weight-loss solution, the diet you can whip out anytime you need a tune-up or when you're looking at another must-look-my-best event on your calendar. The rest of the time, you need to follow a way of eating and moving that you can sustain for life.

The solution: *The Skinny Rules*. There you'll find my twenty nonnegotiable principles, as well as meal plans and recipes that you can adopt as your everyday go-to way of eating. You'll be eating carbs for lunch as well as breakfast, you'll have more daily calories (and a little more salt), and you can go back to eating fruit every day.

*The Skinny Rules* doesn't call for you to have fish oil and electrolyte replacement every day, but if you keep up your exercise routine and/or are exercising enough to sweat, there's no harm—and lots of upside—to continue that part of the Jumpstart program.

Here's what reviewers and fans have been saying about *The Skinny Rules:*

> "I was looking for a system instead of a diet and found this book. I lost 5 pounds in a week, 12 in three weeks, then 5 more pounds for a resounding 20 pounds total soon after. If you have the reason to go for skinny, Bob will give you rules to get there. This book works."
>
> —Dan N., Scotts Valley, California

> "Fans of *The Biggest Loser* already know that supertrainer Bob Harper can transform a morbidly obese couch potato into a six-packed athlete in the course of one sweaty TV season. But can Bob help those of us looking for a no-sweat miracle? The surprising answer: Yes, he can! . . . One little rule. That's all it takes."
>
> —*Woman's World*

> "Harper aims to take the guesswork out of weight loss and set you up for success."
>
> —*Country Living*

"The *Biggest Loser* star has 20 simple ideas—and more than 90 recipes—that help make dropping pounds easier."

—*People*

"The best thing about these rules is that Bob also gives great tips on how you can incorporate these rules into your lifestyle until they become a habit and you no longer need to think about them."

—Sarah, Eastman, Georgia

"After 13 seasons of *The Biggest Loser,* contestants who end up on Bob Harper's blue team probably know what they're in for: a tough-love trainer who will push them beyond what they believe their bodies can do. Now everyone can get a taste of that no-nonsense guidance with Bob's new book, *The Skinny Rules.*"

—*Spry* magazine

"*The Skinny Rules* got me back on track. Other family members have lost weight, too, eating the foods I have been preparing based on this book. Skinny Rules is a healthy way to eat for the rest of your life."

—Linda, Ridgefield, Connecticut

"The author is a great motivational writer and speaker. So, if getting 'the skinny' from Bob Harper is what will help you, then this is the book for you."

—Dan W., San Jose, California

"These are 20 simple rules that will help you change the way you look at food, help make better choices, and lose weight. I got this book the first week it was released and each day I would read a rule and apply it for that day. Two weeks with this book and I already feel a difference."

—Lesia, Statesboro, Georgia

# NOTES

## INTRODUCTION

*when scholars at Laval and Sherbrooke Universities compared:* H Arguin, "Short- and long-term effects of continuous versus intermittent restrictive diet approaches on body composition," *Menopause*, 2012 Aug; 19(8): 870–6.

*Interestingly, a recent study of female military personnel:* GR Hunter, "Exercise prevents regain of visceral fat," *Obesity*, 2010 April; 18(4): 690–5.

## THE JUMPSTART RULES

### Rule 2

*As early as 1995, researchers at the University of Pittsburgh:* RR Wing, "Use of very low-calorie diets in the treatment of obese persons," *Journal of the American Dietetic Association*, 1995 May; 95(5): 569–72.

*"LCD (low calorie diet)-induced changes in BMI [and] fasting insulin":* MH Wong, "Caloric restriction induces changes in insulin and body weight measurements that are inversely associated with subsequent weight gain," *PLoS One*, 2012 Aug; 7(8): e42858.

*And another study, from Maastricht:* WH Saris, "Very-low-calorie diets and sustained weight loss," *Obesity Research*, 2001 Nov; 9 Suppl 4: 295S–301S.

### Rule 4

*In 2010, a group of researchers for the Institute for Public Health:* EA Dennis, "Water consumption increased weight loss," *Obesity*, 2010 Feb; 18(2): 300–7.

### Rule 6

*University of Birmingham researchers studying exercise physiology:* J Achten, "Optimizing fat oxidation through exercise and diet," *Nutrition,* 2004 Jul–Aug; 20(7–8): 716–27.

### Rule 9

*In August 2012, researchers at China's Zhejiang:* SP So, "Screening and identification of dietary oils," *BMC Complementary and Alternative Medicine,* 2012 Aug 31; 12(1): 143.

*New research coming out of the Institute of Medical Science in Aberdeen, Scotland:* P Gray, "Fish oil supplementation augments post-exercise immune function," *Brain, Behavior, and Immunity,* 2012 Nov; 26(8): 1265–72.

### Rule 11

*In a nutshell, investigators at University Hospital Zurich:* I Aeberli, "Moderate amounts of fructose consumption impair insulin sensitivity in healthy young men," *Diabetes Care,* 2012 Aug 28. Epub ahead of print.

### Rule 13

*In one study, a group of Japanese civil servants:* H Matsuura, "Relationship between coffee consumption and prevalence of metabolic syndrome among Japanese civil servants," *Journal of Epidemiology,* 2012 Feb 18; 22(2): 160–6.

*"Dark roast coffee is more effective than light":* C Kotyczka, "Dark roasted coffee is more effective than light roast coffee in reducing body weight," *Molecular Nutrition Food Research,* 2011 Oct; 55(10): 1582–6.

*So says a report from the exercise physiology laboratory at the University of Castilla-La Mancha:* R Mora-Rodriguez, "Caffeine ingestion reverses the circadian rhythm effects on neuromuscular performance in highly resistance-trained men," *PLoS One,* 2012 April; 7(4): e33807. Epub April 4.

# ACKNOWLEDGMENTS

I had so much fun writing *The Skinny Rules* and giving people a list of rules to live by because, let's face it, I love telling people what to do! It felt natural to get the whole band back together to put together *Jumpstart to Skinny*. A huge thank-you to: my writing partner, Greg Critser; my editor, Marnie Cochran; the rest of the team at Ballantine; kitchen guru Danielle Bernabe; my agents Brett Hansen and Richard Abate; my lawyer, P. J. Shapiro; and my right-hand "man," Nicole Trinler.

# INDEX

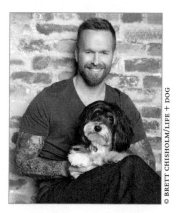

BOB HARPER is a world-renowned fitness trainer and the longest-reigning star of the NBC reality series *The Biggest Loser,* which went into a fourteenth season in January 2013. He has released several popular fitness DVDs and is the author of the #1 *New York Times* bestseller *The Skinny Rules.* Harper still teaches a local spin class in Los Angeles, where he resides with his dog, Karl.

WWW.MYTRAINERBOB.COM

GREG CRITSER is a longtime science and medical journalist. The coauthor of Bob Harper's *The Skinny Rules,* Critser is also the author of the international bestseller *Fat Land: How Americans Became the Fattest People in the World.* He lives in Pasadena, California.

## ABOUT THE TYPE

This book was set in Minion, a 1990 Adobe Originals typeface by Robert Slimbach. Minion is inspired by classical, old-style typefaces of the late Renaissance, a period of elegant, beautiful, and highly readable type designs. Created primarily for text setting, Minion combines the aesthetic and functional qualities that make text type highly readable with the versatility of digital technology.

# THE JUMPSTART RULES

**RULE 1:** Take Control with Proper Proportions—40/40/20

**RULE 2:** Cut Back on Calories. Then Cut Back Again.

**RULE 3:** Eat No Complex Carbs After Breakfast

**RULE 4:** Get Rid of Water Weight by Drinking More Water

**RULE 5:** Get Your Electrolytes

**RULE 6:** Do 45 Minutes a Day of Low-Intensity Cardio, Preferably Before Breakfast

**RULE 7:** Five Times a Week, at Any Time of Day, Do 15 to 20 Minutes of My Jumpstart Moves

**RULE 8:** Cut the Salt

**RULE 9:** Take Advantage of the Restorative Power of Daily Fish Oil

**RULE 10:** Fall Back on Veggies!

**RULE 11:** No Fruit During Week 3

**RULE 12:** Lay Off *All* Booze

**RULE 13:** An Espresso a Day . . . or Two or Three

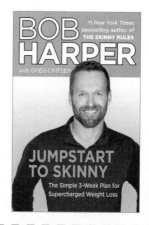

For information address Disney • Lucasfilm Press,
1101 Flower Street, Glendale, California 91201.

Printed in the United States of America

First Edition, September 2015

1 3 5 7 9 10 8 6 4 2

G475-5664-5-15201

ISBN 978-1-4847-2495-8

Library of Congress Control Number on file

Reinforced binding

Designed by Jason Wojtowicz

Visit the official *Star Wars* website at: www.starwars.com.

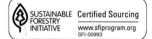